MASTERING MIGRAINE

Finally Understand Migraine, How to Correct its 4 Main Factors and Take Your Like Back!

Dr. Adam Harcourt,
DC, DACNB, FACFN, FABVR

ISBN: 978-1-7333981-9-0 (hardcover)
ISBN: 978-1-7333981-2-1 (audio book)
ISBN: 978-1-7333981-1-4 (epub)

The information contained in this book is the view of the author, unless otherwise stated, and is not intended as direct medical advice. This book is not intended as a substitute for consultation with a licensed healthcare practitioner, such as your physician. Before you begin any healthcare program, or change your lifestyle in any way, it is recommended that you consult your physician or another licensed healthcare practitioner.

Printed in the United States of America.

Dedicated to my incredible wife Mallory. All credit for this book goes to you, as you are the one who made it possible.

TABLE OF CONTENTS

FOREWORD

This book is an easy and informative read. Uniquely, it is a book that has been written for those people that suffer from migraines, and in a style that fits their needs. The flow of the book makes sense as it takes the reader on a logical journey in a logical order with suggestions, models and conclusions that are also logical. Dr. Harcourt includes stories of real patients whose suffering resonates with the reader. At the base of all of it is a glimmering concept of hope for the more than 38 million people in the United States alone and suffer from migraines; and then there is our world.

He attempts to embrace migraine in an evidence based fashion that promotes reasonable concepts that resonate well with a treatment approach suggesting efficacy in its outcome. The reader is taken through a historical journey that involves a simplification of concept theories. Dr. Harcourt presents a rationale for his understanding of the broad field of migraine and contrasts his thoughts with those of others. He makes strong arguments that are persuasive but not so dissimilar from the arguments made by others. His word does stand out, however, because he leads the reader towards a potential hope of beneficial treatment outcomes. He challenges us to take him to task and prove him wrong if we can.

Throughout this book, the reader is exposed to a concept or theory involving the "bucket" or area of the brain that might not be working well. He suggests that identification of this "bucket" might be done by clinicians that have the skills to target this area. He further identifies main contributors that might fill the "bucket" such as dysfunction of hormones, muscles, joints and our individual nutrition. He describes an approach that involves a patient specific rehabilitation that utilizes therapies that do not involve drugs or surgery. All of what he presents does make sense and certainly it entices the migraine suffer to put him to the test to see if what he is saying really works. The manner in which the book is written suggests that there are no side effects to be concerned with by giving his methods a try. Certainly there is hope throughout the read and Dr. Harcourt does a good job of presenting a treatment that is safe and that makes good sense.

The book is refreshing as it does address a variety of potential causes of migraine. The author gives evidence that links migraine to a variety of conditions that may have been passed over during a migraine sufferer's search for relief. It is a short read that is concise in its length without sacrifice of the theme of its content. It is not a textbook that addresses the technical and scientific reality of migraine in a detail that might be a challenge for the average reader. This book should not be considered to be an academic work as there is much that is not said about the subject. But this was not the purpose of the work.

He has convinced me that his thoughts are worth a try. He does not make any outlandish claims, yet shares realistic stories of patients that he has been able to attend successfully. His writing is fluent, understandable and he has done well by taking difficult concepts and reducing them to simplistic themes. As such, this book is one of the few that I think might be read from cover to cover. It certainly is worth the read.

Dr. Frederick R. Carrick

INTRODUCTION

This book is meant both for migraine sufferers and healthcare practitioners. The first few chapters will explain migraine in broad terms to introduce the concepts that are explored later in more detail. It is meant as a summary of what the current research says and my application of that research thus far. If you want to dive more into the 'nitty gritty', I would encourage you to read the last few chapters on genetics, neurological dysfunction, nutrition, hormones, and musculoskeletal stress. If not, simply skip these. If you want to continue to learn even more, I have included references at the end of the book that are sited throughout.

In some chapters you will find that I talk about concepts or ideas about migraine that are not fully cited. This is deliberate, as some of my observations and ideas about the condition are based on the current research as well as observation and have yet to be documented in medical literature. These concepts and ideas are what I hope leads to further discussion and new avenues of research down the line, so if you find a concept that is not referenced it is most likely my opinion or a summary of current knowledge.

This book is not meant as a comprehensive research paper or a way to describe every aspect of migraine. It is intended to combine what has recently come out in research and years of clinical observations treating hundreds of migraine patients. Normally when I speak to other practitioners about what causes migraine, I get answers that vary quite widely. If we can all get on the same page about what is going on with migraine, then the discussion on how to treat it becomes more focused. It also means that there will be research that continues to evolve that will shape and update the opinions expressed in this book. I expect that in the future I can write a second edition that confirms some of my ideas, but also that changes some as well. If there's one thing I've learned about migraine over the years, it's that there is very little about it that's black and white. Both the understanding of migraine and its successful treatment lies in the nuance and customization of care required by each individual patient.

My hope is that by the end of this book you will have the most up-to-date understanding of migraine and what you can do to be in control of this debilitating condition. If you're a patient, I hope that means you can get proper treatment and this book starts your journey toward healing. If you're a practitioner, I hope that it guides your treatment and referrals of each new migraine patient that walks through your door. If you're a researcher, I hope it sparks new questions and queries that will lead to a more comprehensive understanding of migraine in any capacity. I'm also looking forward to the conversations that this book will spark. As with any topic that is not cut and dry, I've found that there is still a fair amount of opinion and dogma that continues to drive these conversations. Ultimately, the better we can understand the altered brain state that is migraine, the better our treatments and outcomes will be.

CHAPTER 1

BACKGROUND

I never expected to write a book about migraine. Growing up I didn't know many people who suffered from the condition and I didn't experience them myself. When I started in the healthcare field almost a decade ago I learned more about it, but basically thought it was a type of bad headache. However, as my education continued and I learned more about the condition and had first-hand experience of treating it, I began to see how much of a problem migraine really was.

On its own, migraine is the sixth most common cause of disability on the planet and the second most common cause of years lived with disability (YLD). (Bonafede, 2017; Burch, 2018.) When you combine migraine with medication overuse headache (MOH, a chronic daily headache and a secondary disorder in which acute medications used excessively causes headache in a headache-prone patient), which is now attributed almost exclusively to migraine medications, it becomes the second most common cause of disability on the planet! The average costs associated with treatment for chronic migraine patients is over $13,000 per year, and those that have tried more than two medications are spending on average $18,000 per year! These costs tend to compound on each other, as many migraine patients tend to get worse over time, miss more work, have less income, and subsequently suffer more attacks. Many patients I've seen have either been unable to work for a certain amount of time or can only work part-time or from home. All of these factors lead the burden of migraine to be almost $20 billion per year in the U.S. alone.

I also began to understand why it is treated, diagnosed, and managed in its current fashion (i.e. not well). This book is meant to give hope and answers to those dealing with migraine, and direction and understanding to those treating the condition. My goal is to help unify the theories and treatment approaches for all practitioners so that no matter what your specialty is, you will have more to offer the next migraine patient that walks through your door.

What really pushed me over the edge, though, was the constant and consistent story that I would hear from people from all over the world. Whether they were in Australia, the U.S., Canada, Iceland, Fiji, or Lebanon, they all dealt with the same progression of migraine that leads to the same progression of treatment. First, they weren't sure if they even had the condition or not. Next, they were given some type over-the-counter medication. Then, as the migraines become more frequent, they were given abortive medications that are designed to stop a migraine once it has begun, such as Triptans. Then, when the migraines became so frequent that they couldn't have any more Triptans, they were given Botox or nerve ablation surgery or any number of other methods. When they still continued to get worse, they were basically told 'sorry, there's nothing else we can do'. I want to highlight the universality of this crisis because there isn't one bad doctor that was just brushing patients off or not listening or not trying. Everything that was thrown at them was based on the current and accepted understanding of migraine, which has led to massive suffering for these people over decades. All of the treatments were addressing the *end* result of migraine, not migraine itself.

While it's amazing that we have medications that can help a migraine once it has started, it doesn't do anything to address *why* the symptoms occurred in the first place. Think of it like this: imagine you are walking down the street and step on a nail. Now you could analyze the fact that inflammatory cytokines are rushing to the area causing inflammation and pain. You could show how the tissue damage and bleeding are leading to the continuation of pain. You could prescribe anti-inflammatories for the cytokines and anti-clotting medications to stop the bleeding, all while ignoring the giant nail stuck in your foot. These methods would technically be addressing the end result of the injury, but wouldn't it make more sense to pull the nail out? Current migraine treatments are attacking migraine in much the same way; eventually you have to look at the nail.

When my wife and I first opened our practice in Santa Barbara, CA, I was focused on managing multiple sclerosis (MS) and traumatic brain injury (TBI). I had just presented a paper on MS at a research symposium and my field of functional neurology was doing a lot with TBI at the time. However, Santa Barbara already had a pretty great TBI rehabilitation center that combined many different modalities. While I could add some value, it wasn't an immediate need in the community. As far as the MS population was concerned, I found that a number of these patients also had migraines. Due to my background in functional neurology and therefore the type of examination that we performed, I began to see patterns that indicated that the MS patients with migraine also had autonomic asymmetry (this will be discussed later in the book).

Thinking that I had made some groundbreaking discovery, I scoured the current research for indications that this had already been established. To my surprise I found many papers discussing the topic, but with very different outcomes. Some papers said that one side of the autonomic system was overactive; the next said it was underactive. Then, other papers would say the same thing about the opposite system.

For example, a paper out of Australia indicated that migraine patients have a local parasympathetic deficit (Drummond, 1997). However, other papers suggested an exaggerated parasympathetic response (Eren, 2018; Avnon, 2004). Yet another supported the idea of sympathetically-mediated hyper-responsiveness in migraine (Wallasch, 2011). Then you have a paper that says there is no difference in autonomic function! However they did conclude that there were only a few tests used and further investigation was needed as all of the tests did indicate a slight tendency toward more sympathetic activation (Rauschel, 2015). This was the beginning of my dive into a new treatment paradigm for migraine. How could there be such a widespread disparity in findings for the same condition? Also, despite all of this information none of the papers offered any suggestions on how to go about treating these new findings.

Patient Story

Mary

Mary had a 20-year history of migraine. When it first began, she would only have about three per year, but over time they progressed. First it was every other month, then once a month, then every other week, once a week, and eventually she was having at least 12 migraines every month. (This is a classic archetype for migraine patients that have been suffering for years.) She was on over 300 mg of Topomax as a preventative and Imitrex when she had migraines, as well as birth control.

As you can imagine, the amount of medication she was taking masked how bad her migraines really were. They were also putting increased stress into her system. While this is common for our patients now, I wasn't aware of how much of a rollercoaster ride we were in for because of the withdrawal symptoms.

Mary improved almost immediately, but continued to have episodes on a reduced yet consistent basis. In addition to there being a number of musculoskeletal and neurological components to her treatment, her hormonal testing showed some of the lowest numbers I had ever seen! We found out that the combination of weaning Mary off medications and the slower process of hormonal treatment, she took longer than expected to recover. After about 2.5 months of on and off treatment, she was able to discontinue all her medication and was experiencing 0–1 migraines/month.

This was a rather challenging case early on, but helped set realistic expectations for a patient so far down 'the migraine spectrum'. She has continued to do well over the last few years and reports having short flare-ups during intense times of physical and mental stress. The best part was that her and

> her family had always wanted to travel oversees for a long stay, but never made plans because of Mary's migraines. Since she was feeling better, they moved to Europe to study abroad for an entire year with their kids!

As I would discover in subsequent years, there is a vast disconnect between what is found in medical literature about migraine and how it is treated. I will discuss an emerging field, functional neurology (also known as clinical neuroscience) and how it is positioned to explain and help treat disorders such as migraine. Those disorders have obvious symptoms, but not-so-obvious causes. I will also discuss how our new understanding of migraine has led me to create a whole new way in which migraine can be viewed and treated. Currently there are over 38 million people in the U.S. suffering from migraines, with more than 4 million having more than 15 every month! The sheer amount of time and money wasted on such a 'benign' condition baffles the mind. It is my hope that creating a new framework in which to view migraine will allow practitioners of any kind to understand not only how they can help migraine patients, but also what their next step should be. Instead of blindly trying different treatments, let's start to address migraine in a systematic, evidence-informed, and effective treatment approach.

CHAPTER 2

WHAT IS MIGRAINE?

Answering the question 'what is migraine?' is ultimately what guides our treatment of the condition. The basis of the most current treatments stems from the school of thought that says that migraine has something to do with aberrant pain signals, and providing pain medications or increasing certain neurotransmitters will fix it. While this does help in the short term, it's only addressing the final result of the entire syndrome that is migraine. It goes back to the analogy of the nail in the previous chapter: why treat the symptoms of having a nail in your foot when you could just pull it out?

In order to understand migraine, we have to understand the concept of functional neurological disorders. Functional neurological disorders are those that present with obvious symptoms but lack obvious pathology. Migraine is a great example as it creates clear and obvious symptoms, but there are rarely any findings upon imaging or with blood work. Other common functional neurological disorders include post-concussion syndrome (PCS), many forms of dizziness, and some movement disorders. This terminology has recently also been used to describe psychiatric conditions, previously known as psychogenic, which is not what is being discussed here.

FUNCTIONAL NEUROLOGY (CLINICAL NEUROSCIENCE)

During the past century, we have made incredible advances in healthcare and medicine. We are able to cure infection with the use of antibiotics, save limbs with cutting-edge surgeries, and even transplant organs from one person to another. With all of these modern advances, the current model of healthcare was born. This model is essentially an emergency or life-threatening medicine model. It uses drugs that can temporarily change physiology in order to stop a wound from hemorrhaging or becoming infected. This model is incredibly useful for things like car accidents, trauma, or aggressive bacterial infections. However, the idea of changing physiology with medication or using surgical intervention for non life-threatening conditions doesn't have the same effect on functional or lifestyle disorders.

Conditions such as migraine, post-concussion syndrome, many forms of dizziness, and movement disorders, are all conditions with debilitating symptoms, but no overt or pathological cause. The majority of migraine headaches (over 99% with a normal neurological exam) do not involve tumors, a stroke, or some sort of obvious defect (Neff, 2005). Many post-concussion patients are told their imaging and blood work is normal, so they should just feel better with rest. Dizzy patients are told not to move too quickly and to take movement-suppressing medication. While the medication can be very helpful symptomatically in the short term, they are doing nothing to address the actual cause of the symptoms.

The reason for this is the fact that these disorders are of a functional nature, not a pathological one (which is where Western medicine shines). Think of it this way: if your computer isn't working properly, you first check the mouse, keyboard, hard drive, etc. If you find that all of those components are working fine, you know it's not a hardware problem and it's probably a software issue. Migraine is a software issue. There is no overt pathology, there is dysfunction in how the brain is working and communicating with itself. If we can appreciate this and understand that neurons (brain cells) are not healthy or dead, but are rather on a continuum of health, we can begin to understand how migraine should be treated.

Clinical neuroscience has been around for decades, but has only become more mainstream as it has impacted professional athletes, Olympians, etc. Frederick R Carrick, A Harvard Medical School trained Clinical Researcher, Professor of Neurology and Senior Research Fellow at the Center for Mental Health Research in association with the University of Cambridge, has pioneered these techniques over the past 40 years. It was the training and insight into the functionality of the brain gleaned from the teachings of Dr. Carrick that have allowed me to make the observations and subsequent treatment options for migraine.

MIGRAINE HISTORY

Accounts of migraine have occurred ever since humans have been recording medical information. Just as long as we have been discussing migraine, its pathophysiology has been debated. The most 'recent' string of debates began around 150 years ago, which tried to figure out if migraine was more of a vascular issue or a neurological issue. This debate has gone back and forth over many years and continues to this day. Out of all of these discussions have come a few consistent viewpoints: the vascular theory, the neurological theory, the neurogenic inflammation theory, and the central and peripheral sensitization theory. While all of these theories do have merit, the challenge has come from that fact that no one simplified theory has been able to explain all the components of migraine.

Take the vascular theory, for example, which has been one of the more pervasive arguments despite a few vital flaws. The vascular theory is the idea that dilation (or enlargement) of extra-cranial arteries, as well as intracranial arteries, produce activation of pain fibers, resulting in a migraine headache. One issue is the fact that the pulsations during migraine do not correlate with heart contractions. The painful sensations are slower than the heartbeat, meaning that the direct contraction or dilation of the blood vessels does not correlate to the pain associated with migraine (Mirza, 2012). There's also the big issue that while some substances, such as vasoactive intestinal peptide (VIP) and nitric oxide, can trigger migraine and dilation of blood vessels, some do not. VIP causes vasodilation of the blood vessels in the head, but does not induce migraine (Rahmann, 2008). Finally, there was also a study that showed that blood vessels in the head do not dilate during spontaneous migraine or change much when given Sumatriptan (Amin, 2013). All of these findings indicate that the vascular theory, while still relevant to migraine, is not the sole cause of the pain.

Some of the other theories that have been posited have merit, but again do not explain the myriad symptoms and findings associated with migraine. Both the 'neurogenic inflammation' theory and the 'peripheral and central sensitization theory' explain some of the phenomenon we see with the condition, but not the entire syndrome. They also don't account for the fact that we see differences in the migraine patient's brain in between attacks, not simply during.

MIGRAINE EXPLAINED

Ultimately, migraine is a genetic predisposition that creates an altered brain state that allows for certain areas of the brain to fatigue or fail, leading to the symptoms associated with migraine. If the area that fails is in the trigeminal nucleus or areas affecting the trigeminal nucleus, the patient will experience head/face pain. If it's in or around the vestibular nucleus, they will experience dizziness. If it's in the occipital cortex, visual symptoms are common. If it affects multiple parts of the brainstem and opposite cortex the patient will have hemiplegic symptoms such as tingling/numbness or weakness. If we can understand the underlying problem of migraine, all of these seemingly disparate types of symptoms can all be treated in a similar fashion. For me, it all began with a relatively simple finding.

What I first started noticing in migraine patients was a difference in autonomic function (such as heart rate and digestion) between those with migraine and those without. I would see things like patients having higher blood pressure on one side versus the other. To understand this, let's take a look at the equation for blood pressure:

MAP = CO × TPR
MAP = mean arterial pressure (blood pressure)
CO = cardiac output (how much blood the heart pumps)
TPR = total peripheral resistance (basically how tight the blood vessels are).

Obviously you only have one heart, so the only way that blood pressure could be different is if the TPR is different from side to side. This can happen when the control mechanisms for the blood vessels on one side are not functioning as well as the other. If there is more activation of the sympathetic (fight or flight) system, the blood pressure will be higher on that side. Conversely, if there is more activation of the parasympathetic system (rest and digest), the blood pressure will be lower on that side.

When I first looked at the research into changes in the autonomic nervous system (ANS) (sympathetic 'fight or flight' and parasympathetic 'rest and digest') with migraine patients, I realized what might be going on. The ANS is primarily controlled by an area known as the hypothalamus in the center of the brain, and then subsequently by many other areas in the brainstem and spinal cord. Ultimately the job of the ANS is to get blood to the area of the body that needs it the most. For example, the sympathetic 'fight or flight' system will shunt blood to muscles and the heart, and away from things like the digestive system. This is an attempt to help the body get away from danger. In contrast, the parasympathetic 'rest and digest' system helps to process food and heal tissues in times of rest. However, there are occasions when you may just want to shunt blood to one side of the body and not the other, so there are areas in the brainstem that control the left or right side of the ANS. This can happen at a few different areas on either side. For example, if I wanted to move my right arm, I would want to activate the sympathetic nervous system to shunt blood to the right arm, but not to the left arm. Therefore, even though there is an overall activation of the autonomic nervous system, there are other 'checkpoints' along the brainstem that inhibit the blood from going anywhere other than the part of the body for which it is intended. Failure of this mechanism can lead to quantifiable changes of the autonomic nervous system from side to side.

This understanding that the ANS can not only be regulated by different levels of the brainstem, but also on either side, led to my first hypothesis. The reason that the research is so conflicted is due

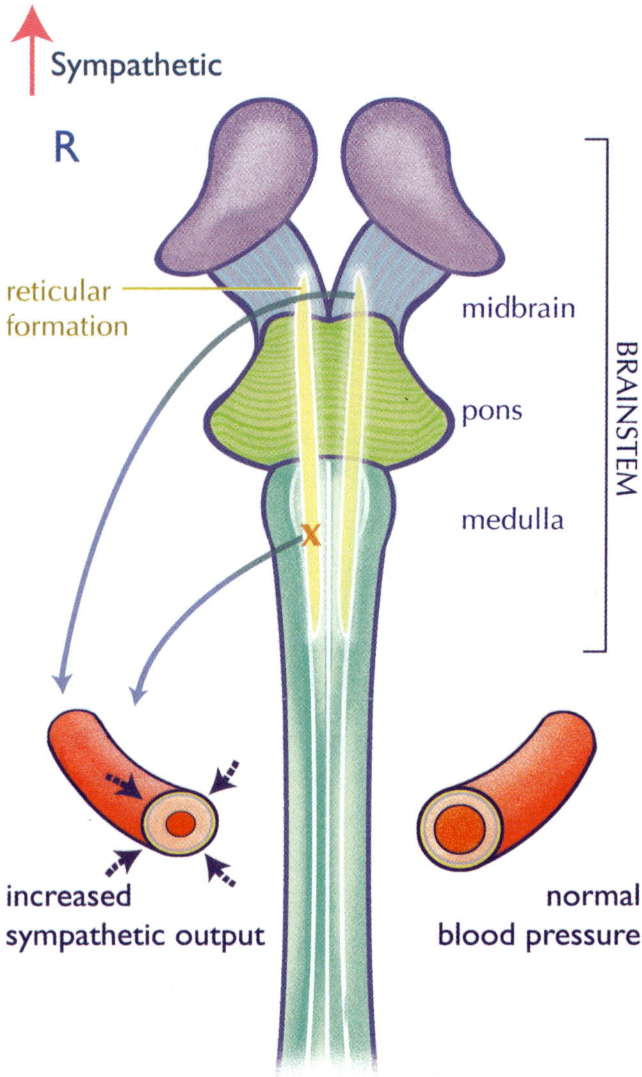

The autonomic nervous system is controlled centrally through the hypothalamus, but also on each side of the body to ensure blood flow gets to the proper area. If any part of the brain or brain stem is not functioning properly, you may not see global autonomic dysfunction, but rather imbalances from side to side. One way to measure this is by looking at bilateral blood pressure. It should be the same from side to side, but a small increase on one side or the other may indicate dysfunction. If there are large discrepancies, however, that may indicate cardiovascular disease.

to different parts of the brainstem being dysfunctional in each migraine patient. This would allow for person A to have an overactive sympathetic system, while person B appears to have an underactive sympathetic system. Therefore, treating all migraine patients with the same therapies would produce different outcomes.

This theme was found in a number of research papers, as cited in the previous chapter. In one paper discussing POTS (postural orthostatic tachycardia syndrome) and migraine, the authors summed it up by saying "migraine patients with accompanying autonomic symptoms seem to experience their pain more unilaterally and more severely than non-autonomic migraine patients … changes in biochemical parameters suggest abnormalities (hypo- or hyper-functioning) of both the sympathetic and parasympathetic nervous systems" (Piovesan, 2008). This was basically what I was seeing. True migraine was accompanied by autonomic dysfunction while patients with migraine without these findings were suffering with some other type of headache. I believe that as we develop more advanced ways to diagnose migraine, we will have to change migraine diagnoses into 'true migraine' and 'migraine-like headache disorders' to distinguish between true migraine and those that are simply not well classified by other means.

My first attempt to test this theory was by targeting the therapies I was already using to one side of the body or the other. Surprisingly, many patients began to get better, which led to the first tenant of migraine treatment: treat every migraine patient as if they are the only migraine patient. There is a relatively simple principle by which you can treat the condition. First, use current research to find out what modalities have the possibility of helping a patient with migraine. Second, perform a thorough examination of the patient that is right in front of you. Third, pair the research and the exam together to decide what, when, where, and how much of a certain therapy – or therapies – have the highest probability of helping that patient.

This may seem like a relatively basic concept, but in the age of evidence-based treatment, many times practitioners fall on one end of the spectrum or the other. Either A) only treating patients with exactly what the available research says, despite what might be happening with that patient or B) ignoring all research and just listening to 'intuition'. Both of these skills are necessary when dealing with a condition that is not black and white. For example, if the best evidence you can find for the treatment of migraine shows that the therapy is effective 50% of the time, what would you do for the other 50%? What do you do if there are other conditions involved? What if they've been on certain medications or hormones or have had surgeries that impact their condition? All of these factors should change the way in which you treat these patients.

When I was first starting on my migraine treatment journey, there was a good amount of research to say that whatever was going on with migraine, it involved the trigeminal system. This includes parts of the brainstem and surrounding structures that control most of the jaw muscles, and more importantly sensation to the face and head. Based on this and my newfound understanding of autonomic dysfunction, we began treating migraine patients with various therapies that stimulated the trigeminal system and areas of the brainstem that controlled the ANS. At first this was getting us great results just by itself! We were very excited and began to get more complicated migraine cases. We went from seeing patients who had three to four migraines a month to seeing patients who were having 10 to 20 migraines a month. It was at this point that I realized that there was a lot more going on.

After researching more and more, I came to the conclusion that migraine is based in neurological dysfunction, but has many other components that make a person more likely to have an attack. The biggest factors, outside of neurological dysfunction, were musculoskeletal, hormonal, and nutritional stressors. There are a number of other things that need to be considered, such as alcohol intake, water intake, sleep patterns and dysfunction, etc., but I typically addressed these components with my patients before I see them in person. Prior to focusing on functional neurology I did a lot of work in the functional medicine realm, so addressing nutritional and hormonal problems is right up my alley. I began treating patients in this new paradigm and we started to see some really great results.

BUCKET THEORY

So what does all this mean? The best way I can sum it up is with my 'bucket' analogy, which will be further explained in the following chapters. Think of the part of the brain that allows for migraine to occur as a bucket. When the bucket is filled up with stressors (musculoskeletal, hormonal, nutritional, sleep issues, stress, dehydration, etc.) and overflows, you get a migraine. Some patients have very 'big buckets', or healthy brainstem areas, and rarely get a migraine. Those with 'small buckets' will get a migraine as a result of almost any stressor. These are the patients who may try a new diet or acupuncture, and it seems that they did nothing to help. It's not that these weren't helpful treatments, it was just that too many other things were filling up the bucket.

One important point to note about the patients we are seeing is that we are about the 10th doctor that they have seen for their condition. Part of the reason that I'm writing this book is due to the fact that I've had the same conversation with hundreds of migraine patients from all over the world, and the story is the always the same. They've tried over-the-counter medications, abortive medications when they have migraine attacks, preventative medications, Botox, chiropractic, acupuncture, diet changes, homeopathy, and sometimes even surgical nerve ablation. This is the average patient that walks through our door, so if the first nine

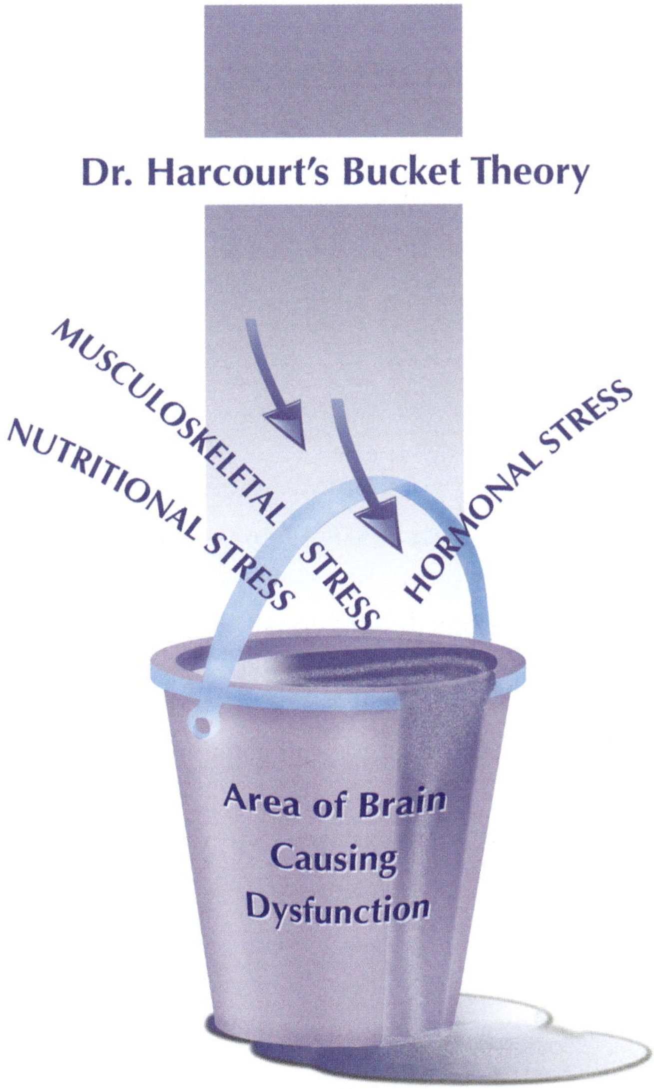

Every migraine patient as an area (or areas) of the brain that are genetically predisposed to have altered excitability. If you imagine those areas as a bucket, when they "fill up" with various stressors and overflow, you get a migraine. Some people have very large buckets, or stable brain areas, so it takes many stressors to lead to a migraine. Some people have smaller buckets, or unstable brain areas, and experience migraine from almost any stressor. Identifying the area of functional deficit in the brain allows us to target therapies or exercises to that part of the brain to stabilize it, or "make the bucket bigger".

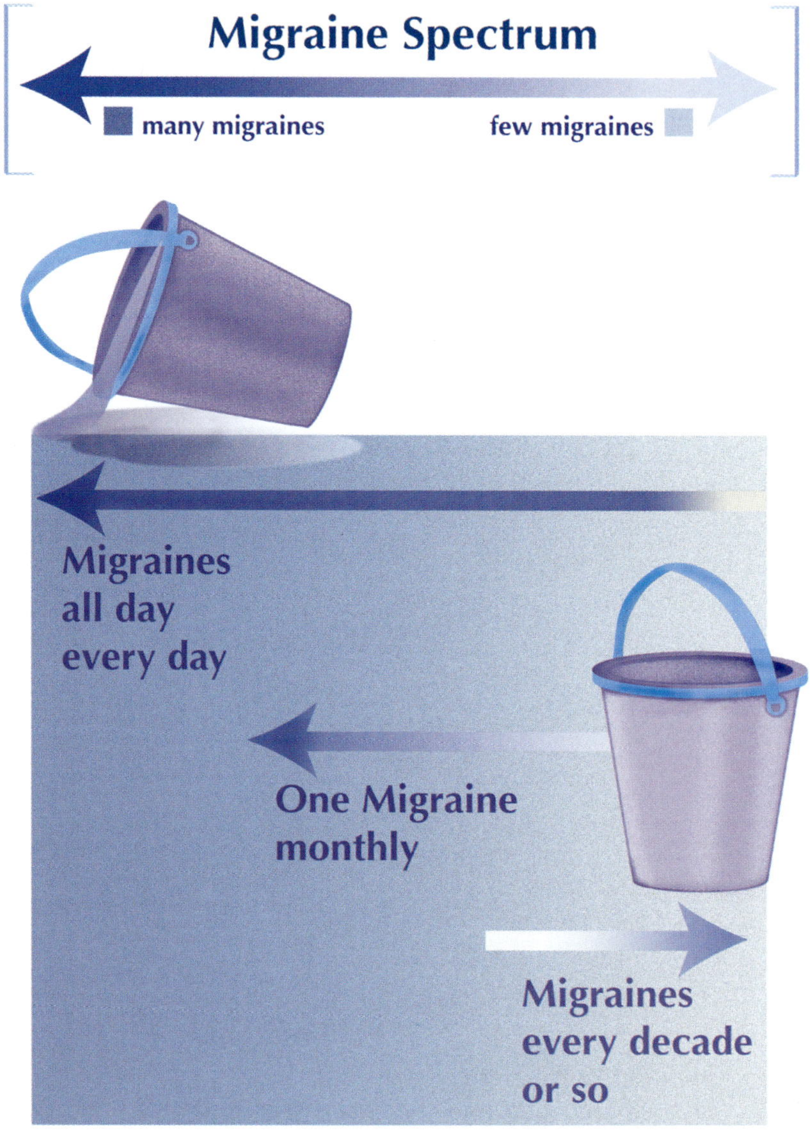

Everyone who has the genetic predisposition for migraine will always have the ability to get a migraine, even if they only get one every decade or so. Depending on the "size of their bucket" and the stressors in their life, all migraine patients are on the "migraine scale". The goal of treatment is to move them down the scale as much as possible to decrease their probability of having migraine.

doctors that they see know the information in this book, hopefully they can find relief much sooner. The key is also understanding that every treatment they received may have actually been helpful, even if they didn't see improvement… it just wasn't the whole story.

So what is migraine? While I'll get into the finer details in the following chapters, migraine is ultimately an altered brain state due to a genetic predisposition. If you are susceptible to migraine, you will always be susceptible to it. However, every patient is on a sliding scale that ranges from those that experience migraines all day every day to those having one only every decade or so. The whole goal with treatment and lifestyle changes is to move you down the spectrum as much as possible. The rest of this book will discuss differing ways in which to do that, and in essence 'make the bucket bigger'.

CHAPTER 3

HOW IS IT CURRENTLY TREATED?

The idea that migraine is an altered 'brain state' is a relatively new idea in the research world and therefore hasn't been incorporated into current treatment protocols. Right now, the main treatments for migraine are focused solely on the end result, which is typically pain. While this is more of a Band-Aid approach to the problem, we also have to realize that it is pretty amazing that there is medicine that can decrease or eliminate an incredibly debilitating condition in a very short amount of time. As with all other treatments, though, these medications must be thought of as piece of the puzzle, and certainly not the full treatment plan.

There are also a number of other options, such as nutrition, chiropractic, acupuncture, massage, etc. that are utilized on a regular basis by migraine patients. The important aspect to understand is that no one treatment is good or bad in itself. Each patient will have different 'deficits' or areas of the brain that need more stimulation, so the acupuncture treatment that works miracles for one person may do nothing for someone else. This is true of all treatments, so the key to proper management is identifying each patient's 'brain state' and assigning treatment accordingly.

Most of the current migraine medications are some type of Triptan. These are a class of medication that are agonists for serotonin receptors. Traditional Triptans affect the 5-HT1B1D receptors, and non-pharmacological or pharmacological prophylaxis is required in patients that have three or more migraine attacks per month (Zebenholzer, 2018). The mechanism of action was originally thought to be due to changes in blood vessels, but newer research is indicating that it may be due to its inhibition of calcitonin gene-related peptide (CGRP) and other pro-inflammatory neuropeptides. There are currently many studies occurring that are developing CGRP antagonists as a new class of drug.

The Triptans and 'abortive' medications are really made for dealing with the occasional migraine when it starts. If you have a migraine every two or three months, it's pretty incredible that you can simply take a medication and not have to deal with it. However, since there is a 'hangover effect' or 'rebound headache' common with these medications, they are not nearly as helpful with chronic migraine. Many of my patients report that on the days that they don't have a migraine, they still feel terrible because they're recovering from the medication taken the day before. We will never tell a patient not to take their medication, as it can alleviate unnecessary pain for many, but most of our patients are anxious to get off of the medication because of its side effects. Clinically, we are seeing that one of the greatest signs of treatment going well is when a patient feels all of the symptoms that normally happen before a migraine, but they don't take their abortive medication and the migraine never occurs. If you understand the 'brain state' paradigm of migraine, you can understand that this means the overall health of the brain and brainstem has reached a level that allows it to stave off a migraine attack. This is an incredibly exciting time for us as we know a patient's long-term outcome is much more promising.

Besides medications to help with the migraine once it's coming on, there are preventative medications as well. There are a few different kinds with varying theories behind why they may work. The most common preventative is the broad-spectrum anticonvulsant drug topiramate, but the mechanism of action is largely unknown. Some recent research has suggested that topiramate may modulate effects of nociceptive processing in thalamo-cortical networks during trigeminal pain (Hebestreit, 2017). I would contend that it is more likely due to the stabilizing of unstable neuronal pools, which is what we see in migraine. However, in migraine there are only certain areas that are unstable and need treatment, which is why patients often complain of many side effects associated with topiramate. Other common preventatives include beta-blockers, calcium channel blockers, tricyclic antidepressants, and selective serotonin reuptake inhibitors (SSRI/SSNRIs). Often migraine patients will go through many different types of preventatives before they find one that works for them, but sometimes none of them will.

Moving to more invasive options, there are surgical interventions that typically involve either the ablation of a nerve or the implantation of a device to continually stimulate the nerve. The most common areas that are ablated or stimulated are the sphenopalatine ganglia associated with the seventh cranial nerve, occipital nerves that that run from the top of the spinal cord up into the scalp, and the trigeminal nerve, which is the largest and most complex of the

12 cranial nerves, through Botox or nerve stimulator. I have had patients report some success with these treatments and others who report none. Knowing that migraine is a 'brain state', nerve blocks serve to decrease input to structures in the brain that have a probability of 'fatiguing' and leading to a migraine. On the other side of the coin, the stimulators make more sense in the brain state model as they strengthen the neuronal pools they fire to. This is why you are seeing more and more devices come on the market that stimulate the nerves in the neck or front of the head. However, if these nerves aren't responsible for most migraines in a patient, either treatment won't help much. There are some practitioners that will 'challenge' these nerves with injections before surgery. That way, if the nerve is involved surgery is indicated and should provide a positive outcome. If the nerve is not involved, the surgery is not performed. While I find that most patients do not need to go to this extreme, I have recommended it for a few for which it was indicated.

In addition to medication and surgical options, many other treatment modalities are utilized by migraine sufferers. They can include nutritional changes, chiropractic, acupuncture, massage, homeopathy, and exercise, etc. I believe that the reason these have all had successful outcomes in certain patients is because they address different aspects of the 'brain state' dysfunction that occurs in migraine. It also explains why there has been no single therapy that has been shown to have consistent and reliable results. When we discuss our approach to migraine, patients discover that many of these therapies are suggested, but only at certain times.

There are also many lifestyle changes that are recommended for migraine patients. Drinking plenty of water, getting enough sleep, avoiding alcohol or caffeine, and regular exercise are all suggested to keep migraines at bay. All of these make sense in keeping with the overall understanding of migraine, but only trying one or two at a time may make them appear to be ineffective. Imagine that your 'bucket' is one-third full from nutritional stress, one-third from musculoskeletal duress, and one-third from hormonal dysfunction. If you just try a new diet, there may be too many other things 'filling up the bucket' to make an impact, so you conclude that diet wasn't helpful. Next, you try hormone treatment because your doctor thinks your attacks could be hormone-related. Again, there isn't much of a change. Finally, you try acupuncture and again there's no change. Individually it looks like each one of these therapies was useless, when in reality they all played a role in you getting better, but they were not used properly. I see this happen so often I'm actually surprised when I find someone who hasn't done all or most of these treatments individually.

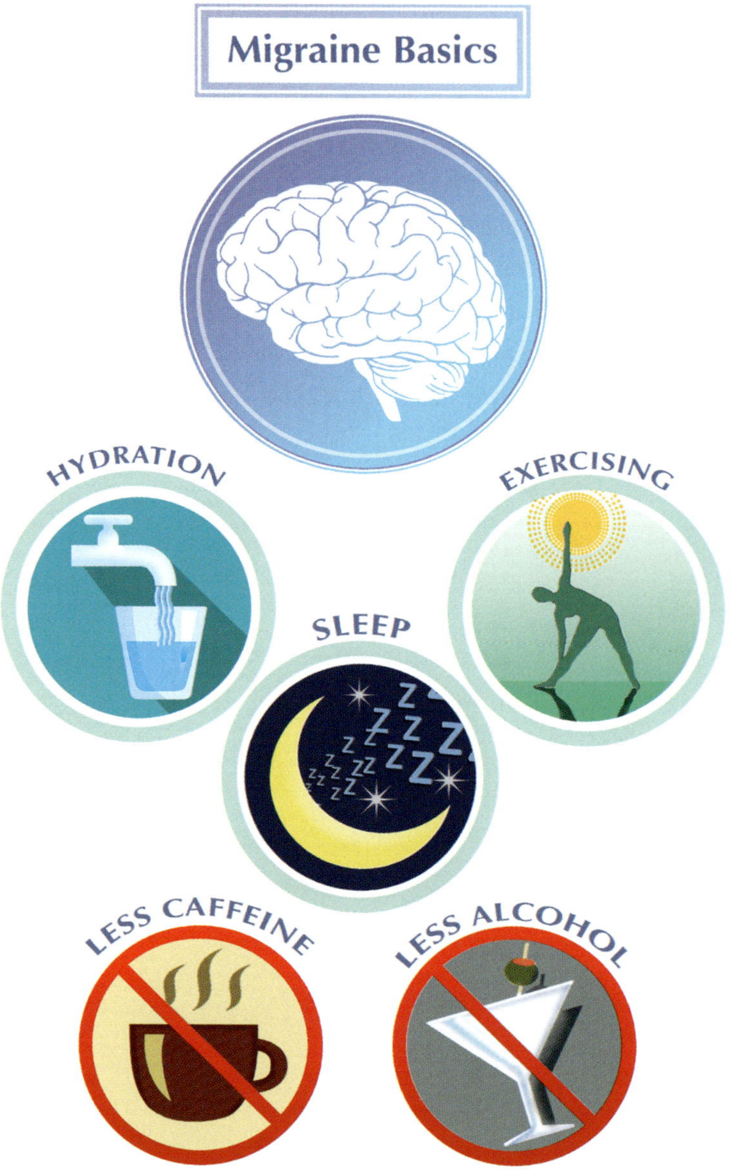

There are many modifiable factors to help reduce migraine, such as proper hydration, exercise, proper sleep hygiene, and reducing caffeine and alcohol. These are all habits that you are able to do on your own and could start today. There are likely many other things to consider for you personally, but addressing these factors are a great place to start.

CHAPTER 4

NEW MODEL OF MIGRAINE

Based on all of the current research as well as my own personal experience with hundreds of chronic migraine cases, the current model and treatment of the condition is significantly lacking. Most patients are treated in a crisis model and deal only with the observable pain and associated symptoms. There is a distinct and real need to start treating migraine for what it is – a chronic disorder that needs to be managed appropriately.

Migraine has evolved over the years to our new current understanding of it as a neurological disorder. When it was first described (and for many years after), it was considered a vascular disorder. Essentially it was thought that the blood vessels would get too big, stimulate the pain receptors in the meninges (the three layers of protective tissue known as the dura, arachnoid, and pia mater covering of the brain and spinal cord), and cause a migraine. Many studies have demonstrated that this is not the case. Another theory is that an attack is caused by neurogenic inflammation in the brain. This mechanism is plausible, but a number of studies have shown that the components of neurogenic inflammation needed for pain are not present in migraine. Also, since migraine attacks can happen frequently over a lifetime, inflammatory mechanisms would most likely leave more visible damage on imaging, but this is not seen.

The most plausible theory/explanation in the last few decades has been a neuro-vascular theory that suggests peripheral and central sensitization of neurons. Sensitization is common in many chronic pain disorders and is thought to be present during migraine. There are a number of findings with this theory that seem to hold weight. For example, central sensitization of trigeminovascular neurons has helped us to understand hypersensitivity and allodynia (a painful response to a non-painful stimulus) that occurs during migraine. However, there are some rather complex reasons that this theory does not explain everything we typically see in an attack.

A new theory understanding of migraine, the 'brain state' theory, has recently appeared in medical literature. I have been describing this type of migraine pathophysiology for the past few years based on my clinical observations and what I was seeing in the literature, describing what I call the 'Bucket Theory'. The interesting aspect of the literature was that individual papers and ideas were hinting toward this concept, but no one had put it all together. There was one paper showing autonomic dysfunction, another showing nutritional components, another showing what factors impact chronicity, yet another talking about hormones, but none of them were talking together. We began putting all the pieces together for treatment purposes and continued to develop our theory as we saw more and more complicated cases. You can imagine how excited I was to read a paper published in 2017 that actually took

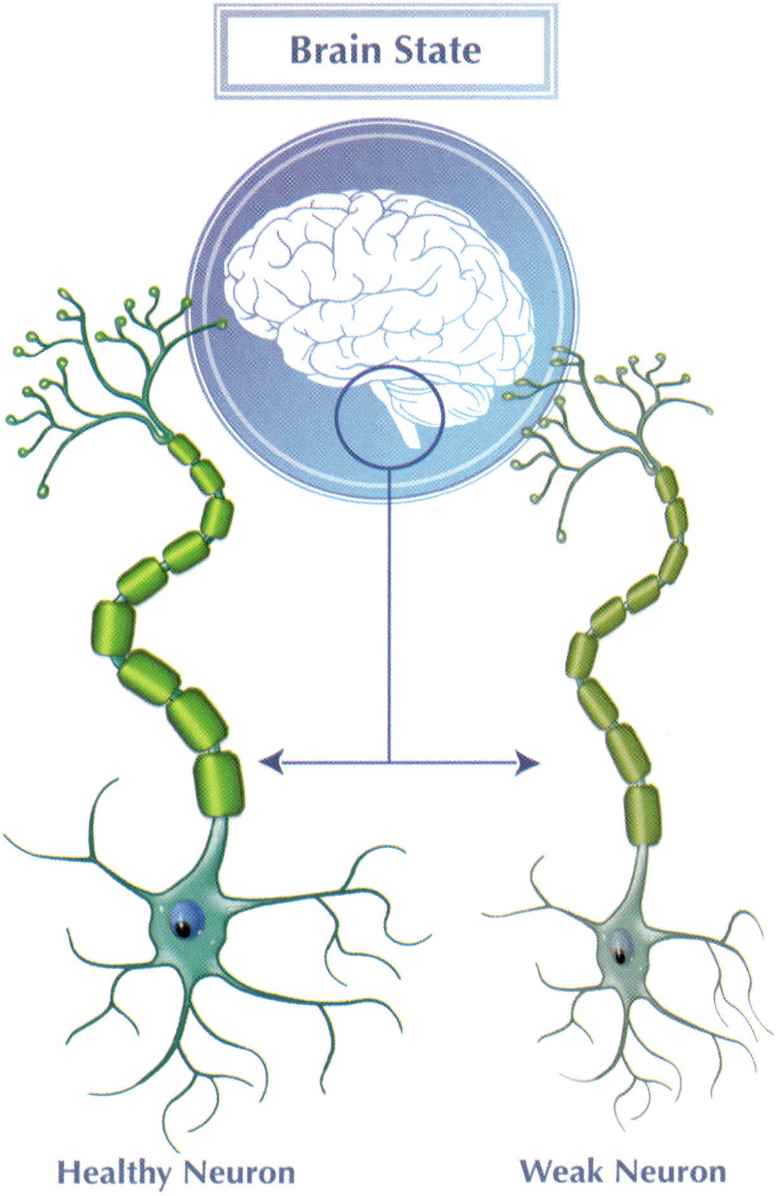

Migraine is an altered brain state, not an obvious pathology that you can see on imaging or in blood work. The neurons that are impacted are not dead or damaged, they are simply not as healthy as the neurons of someone without the predisposition for migraine.

all of the research and came up with a similar conclusion to what I had developed over the past few years!

This model puts the brain at the center of migraine dysfunction, so it is a strictly neurological theory. The brain of a migraineur is functionally different than those who do not have the condition. The experience of migraine occurs when there is dysfunction in the brain, brainstem, hypothalamus, or thalamus. When these areas fatigue or fail, you end up with a migraine. The next step in treatment, which is what I've been working on for the past few years, is to identify the specific areas that are dysfunctional in each individual patient and provide treatments or therapies to strengthen those areas. This isn't a medical or nutritional or chiropractic or exercise-based method, it's a rational clinical approach to a disorder that is different for each person.

One of the most challenging aspects of integrating this new concept into clinical practice is teaching individual practitioners to treat migraine for what it is, and not based on what their specialty is. This is not specific to any type of practitioner, it is universal. If you're dealing with migraines and you go to a medical doctor, you'll get medication. If you go to a chiropractor, you'll get your spine adjusted. If you go to a nutritionist, you'll change your diet. If you go to an acupuncturist, well… you get the idea. It's very important to note that all of these approaches and treatments can absolutely benefit migraine attacks, but they only address specific parts of the disorder and are not a comprehensive approach. This is why your friend will tell you that you HAVE to try this new diet to fix your migraines, because that's what worked for them. All this should be telling you is that your friend had certain dietary components that were the major contributor to their migraines. Are there other things they could do to get even better? Probably. Will the exact same thing work for you? Maybe. You won't know until you try because each person has a different presentation of migraine.

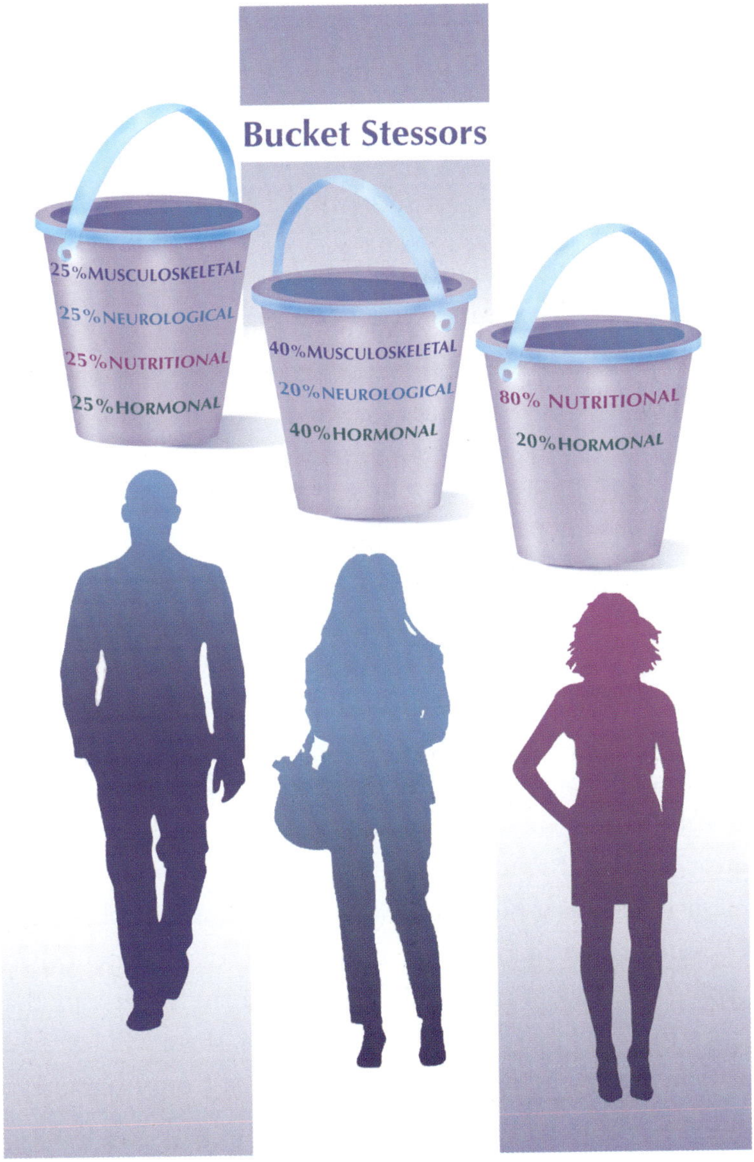
Bucket Stessors
25%MUSCULOSKELETAL
25%NEUROLOGICAL
25%NUTRITIONAL
25%HORMONAL
40%MUSCULOSKELETAL
20%NEUROLOGICAL
40%HORMONAL
80% NUTRITIONAL
20%HORMONAL

Each person will have a different weighted response to each potential stressor. If your "bucket" is filled up primarily by nutritional stressors (high weight), then a new diet may look like a miracle cure. If nutrition doesn't cause that much stress on your system (low weight), it may look like diet doesn't impact you at all. The important part to remember is that everyone is different and must be treated accordingly.

For me it's always been very simple: if we completely understood what was going on, we could provide the perfect treatment and patients would get better 100% of the time. Since that hasn't happened yet, I continue to explore and consider all different types of therapies for migraine, as long as they make sense in 'brain state' model. I even tell many of my patients that the treatment they are getting now is much better than that of my patients a year ago, but not as good as my patients will get two years in the future. All this is to say is that we are continually updating and changing our treatment approaches based on new research and clinical observations.

The most important part of the model, however, is individualized care. Each migraine patient will have different parts of their brain that have genetically altered levels of excitability. The fact that this can happen in multiple different areas of the brain and to differing degrees of dysfunction means that not only do we need to use different therapies, we need to use them in the appropriate amount. There is debate about things like exercise and migraine, for example. Some people say that it's good for migraine; some say it's bad. If your 'bucket' is really small, then exercise may be more stimulation than you can handle. However, that exercise may be great for you if you just start out a little less intense. Unfortunately it is seen as a black and white/all or nothing phenomenon that would cause this person to move on to try a different therapy, bypassing one that was actually great for them. If we can change both doctors' and patients' view of migraine, there will be a radical diminishment in the disability that is created from migraine. This is ultimately what I am hoping to accomplish with this book.

CHAPTER 5

BUCKET THEORY

If much of what I have been describing so far hasn't made a ton of sense to you, I think a return to the 'bucket theory' will clear up any confusion. As I was first developing our migraine program, I was having a really tough time explaining how comprehensive our treatment approach was and why it was different from everything else. At the time I didn't have a whole lot of recognition in my field – no books or affiliation with a prestigious institute, so why should someone entrust their care to me? After a few weeks in a row of being exhausted from trying to explain this time after time, I somewhat accidentally explained it to a patient with a simple analogy: "Having a migraine is like filling up a bucket, it's not until the bucket overflows that you have a migraine, but many things can fill up that bucket."

As we established in the last chapter, there are many different parts of the brain that can be affected in migraine patients. These

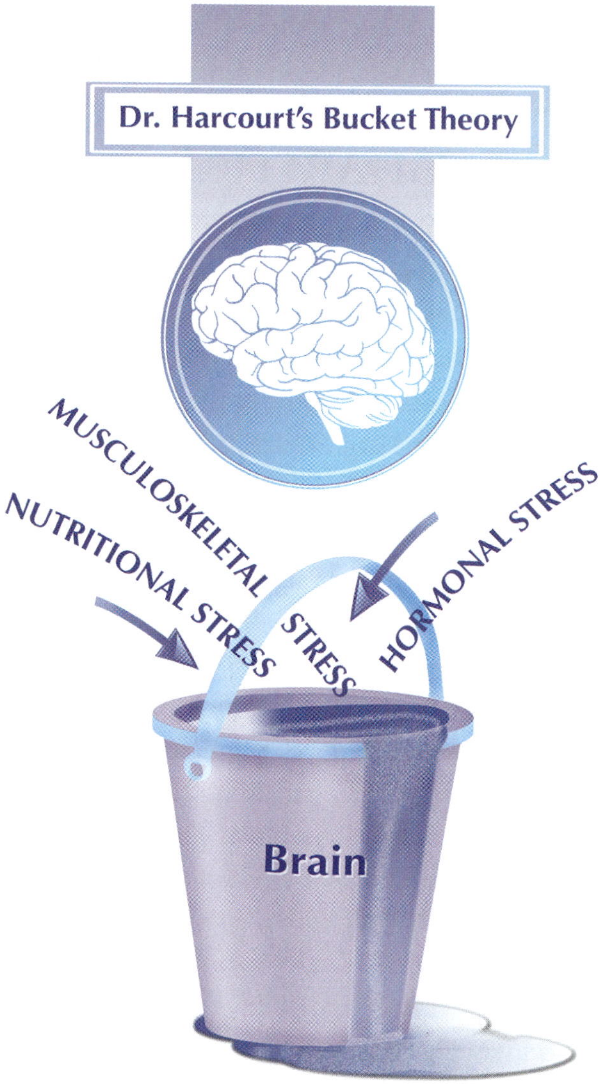

Every migraine patient as an area (or areas) of the brain that are genetically predisposed to have altered excitability. If you imagine those areas as a bucket, when they "fill up" with various stressors and overflow, you get a migraine. Some people have very large buckets, or stable brain areas, so it takes many stressors to lead to a migraine. Some people have smaller buckets, or unstable brain areas, and experience migraine from almost any stressor. Identifying the area of functional deficit in the brain allows us to target therapies or exercises to that part of the brain to stabilize it, or "make the bucket bigger".

areas have the ability to 'fail' and lead to the symptoms associated with the condition. For most migraine patients, this is head/face pain, for some it's ocular symptoms, and for others it can be a sensation of dizziness/vertigo. While the variations are wide, the underlying pathology is the same. Since migraine patients have specific parts of their brain that can become fatigued and fail due to having an altered 'brain state', when they fail that person will get a migraine.

Patient Story

Patricia

Patricia is a 41 year old with a lifelong history of migraines. She reports having them when she was a child, mainly coming on when she was stressed. When we saw her, she was having more than 20 migraines a month. She also reported that she frequently got nocturnal migraines that would wake her up at night. She was on multiple different medications and had tried every diet and exercise routine she could find.

There were two major factors contributing to the progression of her condition. First, she was over-exercising to the point that she told us she worked out for three hours before her first visit! That was after a trip across the country the day before. Second, she only ate once or twice a day, and did not have her first meal until mid-afternoon. Just getting her exercise and dietary regimen under control immediately made a huge difference.

During her examination we found that she had extremely aberrant eye movements in many different directions. We were only able to see her for five days before she flew back home, but we were able to normalize most of her eye movements in a very short time. She also only had one migraine during treatment, which subsided shortly after it came on, and she was surprised as this had never occurred without an abortive.

About a month and a half after intensive treatment, we followed up with her. She reported that she had experienced one flare-up when her husband was sick and she lost a lot of sleep and was not keeping up with the therapies I had recommended for her to continue at home. When she got back on track, she reported no symptoms and was back at work full-time without any medications!

This leads us to two very important concepts when it comes to migraine treatment. First, just because a treatment or therapy didn't show you noticeable changes when you tried it, that doesn't mean it wasn't a good therapy. Second, the therapies that are applied can be great, but they can also sometimes be too much. If you tried exercise and it made you worse, it's probably not the exercise that's the problem, it's probably the amount. Same goes for physical therapy, chiropractic, massage, etc. These modalities can be very powerful, so a little bit goes a very long way. We know that patients are doing extremely well when they can handle any of these treatments without having any type of flare-up. This lets us know that their 'bucket' is growing.

I therefore have two primary goals when treating migraine patients. The first is to identify 'the bucket' or area of the brain that is dysfunctional in a patient. Once we identify the part of the brain that is not as healthy as it should be, we can then provide treatments and therapies that target and strengthen the area, thus 'making the bucket bigger'. The second goal is to decrease or eliminate 'bucket fillers'. The three main contributors, or 'bucket fillers', are nutritional dysfunction, musculoskeletal dysfunction, and hormonal dysfunction. If you can grasp this simple concept, you already have better control over your migraines. If you're a practitioner and can grasp this concept, you are already providing better care to your patients.

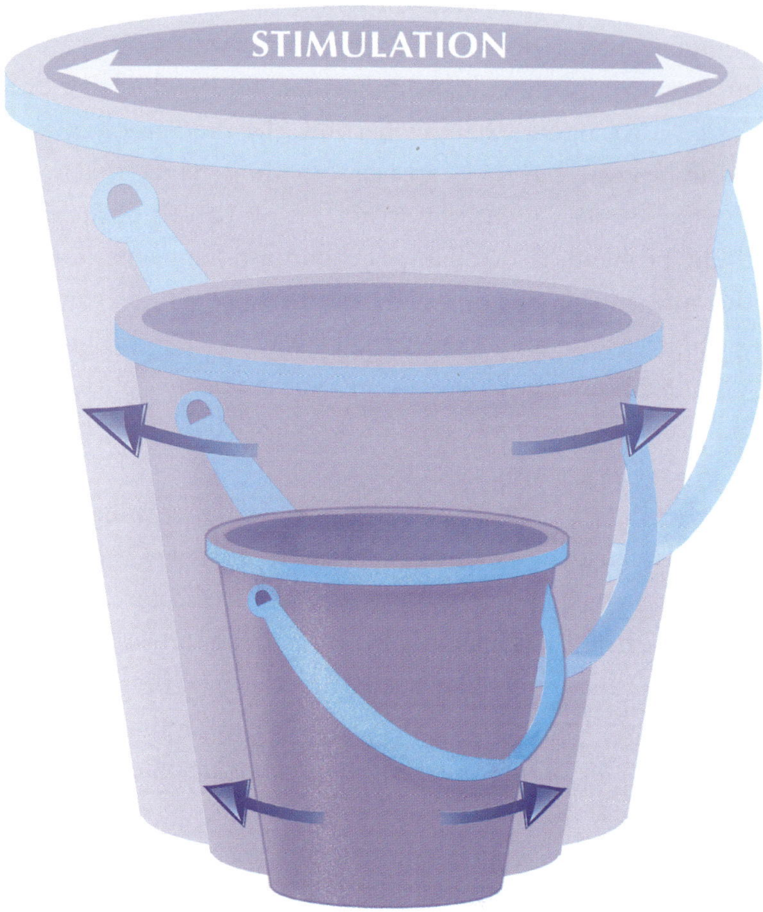

The 'Bucket' Growing with Customized Brain Rehabilitation & Therapies

The altered excitability in the neurons in specific areas of the brain in migraine patients is what can be stabilized to decrease the probability of migraine. One way to do this is through stimulation of those neurons, which produces more protein, which lowers the neuron's resting membrane potential. The further away from threshold the neuron gets, the lower the probability it will fail and cause migraine. The more stable the neurons become, the bigger their "bucket" is.

CHAPTER 6

CONCUSSION & MIGRAINE

Due to the debilitating nature of migraine, and the hopelessness that is generally portrayed to most migraine patient who have 'tried everything', it has been our mission from the beginning to get our message out to as many people as possible. This includes taking time to talk with anyone on the phone who is curious about what we are doing. It has been my privilege to speak with people from all over the world about our treatment approach and simply explain migraine to them. I've gotten feedback on more than one occasion that just understanding what the heck is going on has helped people to reduce their stress levels and ultimately their migraine episodes.

However, one of the reasons I decided to write this book is due to the fact that I often find myself sounding like a broken record.

Many of our treatments have either been developing over time and we are working on researching on a larger scale, or have been taken from current research and applied more specifically for each patient. However, we do this every day for many patients therefore it doesn't seem so strange or different to us. So by the time I talk to the seventh person in a day and am explaining the 'bucket theory' to them, it can be tough to still be excited about it. This book is a way to disseminate this information more efficiently.

Chatting with hundreds of people from around the world definitely had its upsides though. One of the main benefits was hearing the patterns of events or lifestyle habits of many different people. A consistent finding that kept coming up was reports of a concussion or some type of head trauma. It was almost like clockwork that every other person I talked to had a consistent recollection of a trauma preceding their onset of, or massive increase in, migraine.

This leads me to the 3 most common outcomes of concussion and migraine. After a patient has a concussion, there are 3 common outcomes that we commonly see:

1. The patient previously suffered from migraine, but after the concussion they became more frequent
2. The patient did not previously suffer with migraine, but was diagnosed with migraine after the accident since it fits the diagnostic criteria. This situation almost always leads us to find it was post-concussion/traumatic headache without actual migraine.
3. The patient had a genetic predisposition to migraine, but it hadn't yet manifested. The concussion was enough of a trauma to allow the phenotypic expression of their migraine predisposition.

3 Common outcomes with "migraine" after concussion

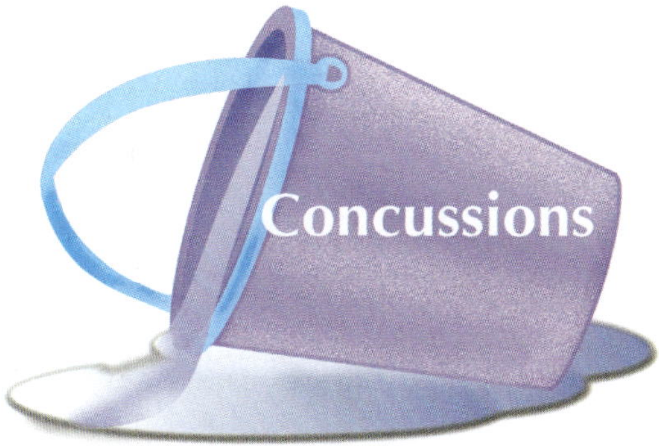

1) They previously had migraine and it gets worse.

2) They didn't have migraine, but after the concussion were diagnosed with migraine, even though it wasn't true migraine.

3) They had a genetic predisposition for migraine and the concussion was enough to "fill up the bucket" and lead them to start having migraine.

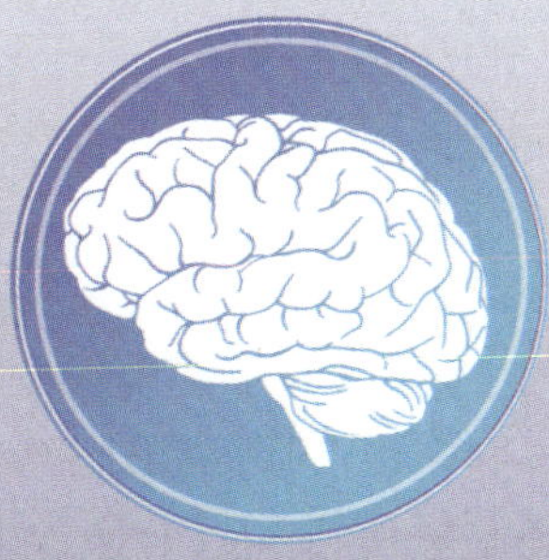

TIME OF CONCUSSION TO ONSET OF MIGRAINE

Now when I say concussion, it's important to note that this doesn't have to involve a hit to the head. Concussion can occur from a whiplash-type injury, such as in a car accident. So when I would speak with patients, there was a high probability that prior to the onset of migraine, there was a concussion or car accident or some type of head trauma about 18–24 months prior. If it was a significant trauma, that time frame could be reduced a bit. I would always get a stunned 'how did you know?' response as frequently these events are not correlated.

As discussed in previous chapters, our new understanding of migraine has to do with the idea that it is a whole brain phenomenon, but there are certain areas of the brain and brainstem that will be more impacted for each patient. The most common areas are located in the brainstem, specifically areas such as the periaqueductal gray, rostral ventral medulla, and locus coeruleus (Goadsby, 2017). The reason that this is important is due to the fact that most of the damage caused by concussion is to, or close to, these parts of the brainstem. The nervous system is driven by electricity, so any area that is stimulated will have an impact on the surrounding structures. Think of it as if you were to throw a rock into a pond. The biggest impact is where the rock lands, but there is a ripple effect all around it. The areas directly adjacent to the rock will be most affected, and that effect will degrade as you get further away from where the rock impacted the water.

This is how concussion impacts migraine. The areas of the brainstem that are damaged from the concussion are already 'weaker' from the person having migraine. The concussion furthers this dysfunction, making their 'buckets' smaller. Therefore, it will take less and less stress in order for that person to have migraines. There is a concept known as diaschisis that helps to explain why it takes time for a head injury to really impact migraine. Diaschisis is defined as "the changes of structural and functional connectivity between brain areas distant to the lesion" (Carrera, 2014). Any area that is connected to the damaged area will begin to show impairment over time due to the lack of activation. So if neuron A supplies neuron B and C, and neuron A dies off, neurons B and C are now getting less activation, and over time will begin to show signs of damage as well.

Patient Story

Margaret

Margaret had a long history of migraines, but had not experienced many in the last few years. She said that chiropractic care had drastically reduced her migraines to a point that they weren't much of an issue, and she would simply take an Excedrin when she did get one. However, two weeks prior to seeing us, she said that she got the worst migraine of her life and it hadn't gone away. She also said that she was extremely dizzy and 'foggy'. She denied any trauma or car accident had recently occurred.

Her examination looked very much like a post-concussion case, so we again asked her if she had any recent trauma and again she said that she hadn't. Based on her examination, we decided we were going to treat this more like a concussion, even though there hadn't been one. To be sure, we also included hormonal and nutritional treatment consistent with migraine care.

After the first few days of treatment, Margaret was no longer experiencing any of the symptoms she presented with. When she went back to work, she found that it wouldn't take too long before she became fatigued and her symptoms would creep back. We worked with her and give her incremental, increasingly challenging exercises until she could get through a full day with no issues.

During one of her follow-up visits, she came into the office with a broken pair of sunglasses. She told us that we'd never believe what happened. She had found a broken pair of sunglasses on the floor of her garage and recalled what happened. About two weeks prior to her symptoms appearing, her garage door dropped onto her head so hard that it broke her sunglasses

> and dazed her to the point that she forgot the incident even happened! She said she now remembered stumbling into the house and resting, but by the next day had completely forgotten that the incident occurred. Luckily her examination had previously clued us in to something like this happening, but we finally had an explanation as to why everything occurred the way that it did. Had we treated her as a 'normal' migraine patient, her case may have progressed very differently.

The good news is you have billions and billions of neurons, so if you lose a few – or even a few hundred – you may never notice. However, if this continues over time without proper treatment, you can see how one or two years down the road you would start to notice the effects of diaschisis. This is why we specialize in post-concussion syndrome as well as migraine, as they go hand-in-hand. Even if you haven't had a concussion, many of the treatment modalities that would help rehab a concussion are extremely effective in treating migraine. I can't tell you how many people I've talked to that have been diagnosed with migraine that actually had post-concussion headaches. This leads to improper treatment and long-term effects that should have been addressed right away. One of the main reasons that this happens is due to migraine and post-concussion syndrome sharing many of the same symptoms. Another reason is due to the lack of objective testing to properly diagnosis migraine or post-concussion.

TESTING

Currently, there is no gold standard in concussion assessment. Concussion (or mild traumatic brain injury, mTBI) by definition is head trauma without any signs on imaging, so when people say that they're fine because their computed tomography (CT) scan was clean, they're really saying that they don't have a traumatic brain injury (TBI). This is great news by itself, because we know that there isn't a brain bleed or swelling, but if a patient is still experiencing symptoms it can be unbelievably frustrating. I can't tell you how many of my patients have been told, "you're just making this up", or "you should be better by now", or "it's all in your head". To say that post-concussion symptoms are psychogenic and have no factual basis is insulting to the patient and devastating to long-term outcomes.

Another reason that testing is important is because it's very clear that the sooner you begin treatment, the more likely you are to recover (Lawrence, 2018; Grool, 2016; Majerske, 2008). If testing is inconclusive or based solely on imaging and the patient is told simply to rest until they feel better, treatment may be delayed by weeks or even months! A few days of rest are fine, but becoming active or undergoing treatment as soon as possible makes recovery much more effective.

While there currently isn't a gold standard for concussion diagnosis, based on research and years of experience many functional neurologists can tell if you've had a concussion simply by looking at the way your eyes move or how well your balance or gait patterns are. Since this takes years of training, I have found a few objective, peer-reviewed methods of assessment that work very well in identifying concussion.

One investigation, developed by a research team at the University of Pittsburgh, uses vestibular/ocular testing as a way to identify concussion, known as VOMS (Mucha, 2014; Yorke, 2017). This method involves using different types of eye and head movements to determine whether or not there has been a concussion. Follow-up studies using this method indicated that a positive VOMS indicated an increased 'return to play' time for athletes (Anzalone,

2017). The reason this type of testing works so well is due to the fact that most trauma arising from concussion occurs in the midline structures of the brain, which are responsible for balance, posture, and eye movements. This makes them easy to assess, but difficult to fake.

There is also a balance platform, or posturography, that we use that can assess concussion based on balance. The reason that I prefer these methods over some of the other more well-known tests is due to the fact that you can't really fake these tests. If you're asked to do a task that involves reflexes you get a better window into the nervous system, as opposed to asking cognitive questions or something that a patient could intentionally or unintentionally falsify. Luckily this phenomenon has been identified and there are measures in the testing protocols that attempt to identify intentional 'sandbagging', but it is something that needs to be considered (Erdal, 2012). Now you might think, "who would fake a concussion test, wouldn't you want to know?" Well, if you're asking that question, you've never met a competitive athlete. It's amazing to me that people would prefer to keep playing their sport and risk their health rather than take some time off, but it's very consistent across all sports, which brings me back to why I like reflexive testing.

Once we have determined whether or not we think someone is having post-concussive or post-traumatic headaches and not migraine, we can begin treating them. I find that there is less reliance on diet and hormonal testing in general with concussion patients vs. migraine patients, so I can start treatment much sooner with concussion patients. This is due to the fact that before I see migraine patients from out of town, I want to have them on a strict dietary regimen for at least a month or so before we meet. This also allows time for hormonal testing and detoxing off of any foods that they might be sensitive to. With concussion patients, most of the cause of headache is neurological, so the sooner we can start treatment the better.

As far as treatment goes, we are using a model similar to the one outlined in a paper from 2017 that involves treatment over a one to two week period in which we can see patients multiple times per day (Carrick, 2017). We have transitioned more to this model for managing concussion over the years as it allows us to make changes to our treatment protocol within hours rather than days. The nervous system and neurons are able to change and adapt quickly, so if we overstimulate the patient, we can change the frequency or intensity of the therapy to make sure it is appropriate. This allows us to make the greatest amount of change in the shortest amount of time.

We re-evaluate the patients every other day to make sure we are being as efficient as possible. By the end of the week, we can give them exercises or a rehab prescription that they will continue at home in order to keep improving their condition. While there is still no treatment that is 100% effective, this method has shown vast improvement in patients that have not benefited from other methods. Just as with migraine, I expect that as more and more research comes out, this type of treatment will become more refined and more predictable in order to better serve these patients.

Chapter 7

Dizziness & Migraine

Dizziness is beginning to be more commonly recognized with migraine. Many of our patients will express feelings of disorientation, spinning, light-headedness and other forms of what is considered dizziness. Some of these sensations can be directly linked to the migrainous state, while others are a separate cause that simply make the patient more likely to have a migraine.

There are many current studies that are linking dizziness and vertigo to migraine. There are also studies that indicate that dizziness and motion sickness improve with various types of migraine medication, including beta-blockers, calcium channel blockers, tricyclic antidepressants, and anti-epileptic drugs (Lee, 2018). There is another study that shows that dizziness and nausea is a common side effect of anti-migraine medications (Gonzalez, 2018), and this one is not alone. There is also a form of the condition called vestibular migraine (VM) that sometimes manifests only as dizziness with no head pain. A recent study looking at eye movements showed that slower total eye speed could be suggestive of vestibular migraine (Thompson, 2017). A separate study showed that recurrent dizziness symptoms brought on by visual or postural motion are predominant in VM patients. Another study showed that the balance of VM patients is altered compared to healthy individuals (Balci, 2018). There is even a study that shows that there can be vestibular alterations in migraine patients who have never experienced dizziness or vertigo (Bernetti, 2018)! These studies are all steps that start to piece together how dizziness and other symptoms that do not seem related to migraine are actually all part of the same disorder.

Vestibular migraine is also likely under-diagnosed in the population of patients that only experience dizziness without migraine head pain or other associated symptoms. A recent epidemiology study indicated a prevalence of VM in 2.7% of the adult population – much higher than previously suspected. Of those patients that met the criteria for vestibular migraine, only 10% were told that migraine was the cause of their dizziness (Formeister, 2018)! A study performed in an outpatient neurological clinic actually put VM as the third most common cause of dizziness in patients under 60 years of age (Pan, 2018). In my opinion, vestibular migraine is simply the amplification of common dysfunction in migraine. We've seen that most migraine patients have some type of subclinical abnormality of their vestibular pathways. In most people, this still ends up manifesting as head pain, with the vestibular dysfunction contributing to the fatigue, or 'filling the bucket' of the trigeminal pain pathways. However, if your primary dysfunction is in the vestibular pathways, the symptoms will manifest as dizziness. I view this as an accentuation of normal dysfunction in migraine, with little dysfunction in other areas of the brain normally associated with the condition.

If we understand that migraine is an altered brain state, and that altered brain state allows certain areas of the brain to have an altered central integrated state (CIS, see chapter 8), it's easy to understand how migraine could affect an area such as the vestibular nuclei in a similar fashion as it affects the trigeminal nucleus. If a person with migraine has most of their dysfunction in the area of the brainstem that helps coordinate where they are in space, and that area fails, you will have an experience of motion or dizziness. We know that there are many areas in the medulla (where the vestibular nuclei are mainly located) that are affected in migraine, such as the nucleus raphe magnus and the rostral ventromedial medulla. As described previously, if an area of the brainstem is stimulated, the areas surrounding it will also have some level of stimulation, the way a rock will produce ripples on water far away from where it lands. If there is dysfunction in the medulla from one area being dysfunctional, there is now a probability that other areas of the medulla will experience dysfunction.

I believe this altered brain state principle of migraine explains vertiginous migraine. When the vestibular nuclei can no longer do its job, it fails and produces the symptoms of dizziness. This is what I think we're seeing in the medical literature, a strange occurrence of vestibular abnormalities and migraine association without a guiding theory to connect the two. The research that indicates migraine patients have subclinical alterations in the vestibular pathway is a window on to the type of dysfunction we have been seeing for years. This helped me to understand that the oculomotor and vestibular aberrancies that we see in our practice every day are in fact indicative of migraine, not just an incidental finding. By correcting or improving the function of these areas, we see continual and steady improvements in the patient's symptoms. I believe the brain state theory explains not only how dizziness can occur through functional failure of the vestibular nucleus, but also how dizziness and migraine are directly related.

An important point to note is that this theory applies to patients with dizziness directly related to migraine. There is also the subject of peripheral vestibular problems leading to an increase in migraine. The most common form of peripheral vertigo is benign paroxysmal positional vertigo, or BPPV. This form of dizziness is believed to be caused by calcium carbonate crystals that fall into vestibular semicircular canals and stimulate the hair cells that detect rotational motion. These crystals are normally located in a different part of the vestibular apparatus and are thought to enter the canals accidentally, most commonly in the posterior canal. The majority of patients with BPPV report that they feel the room start spinning when they lie back at the hairdressers or dentist or in bed. There are simple maneuvers that you can do to fix this in a two to three minute window, but many people are not aware of the maneuver or how to do it properly.

How does this relate to migraine? If we know that the areas around the vestibular nucleus are prone to failure and can lead to migraine, if you overstimulate the vestibular nucleus you're more likely to have a migraine. This goes back to the bucket model, where an overstimulation of the vestibular nucleus is one more thing that can fill up the bucket. The BPPV by itself does not cause migraine, but it does make a patient more likely to have a migraine by making the bucket a little bit 'fuller'. This is why we address peripheral vestibular function in everyone that we treat for migraine. It's not the cause, but it can definitely be a contributor.

Another more common cause of stress in migraine is what we call a central vestibulopathy. Recently it is also being referred

Dizziness

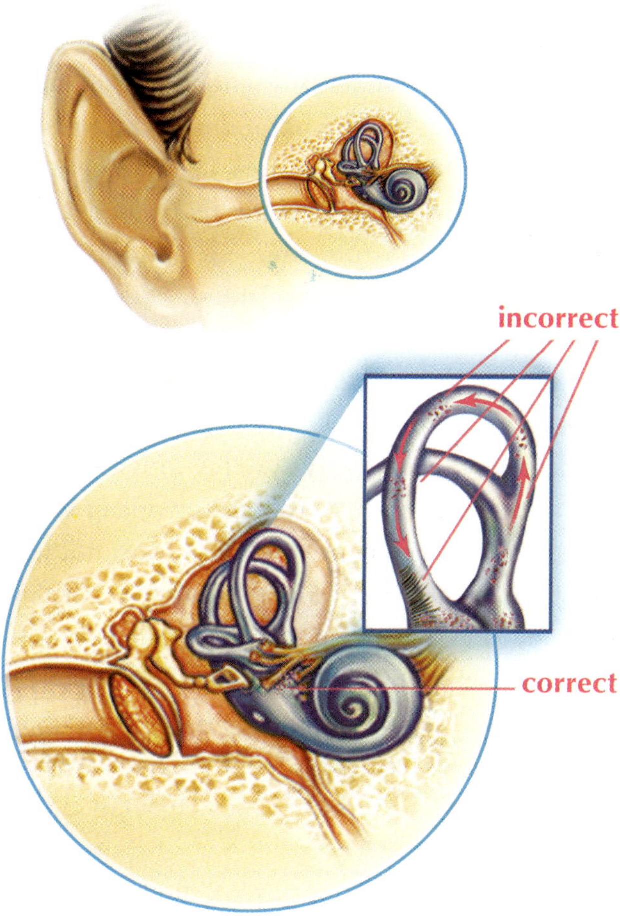

There are many different causes for dizziness. In this example, the patient is suffering from benign paroxysmal positional vertigo, or BPPV. There are little crystals, or otoconia, in part of the inner ear that help detect translation motion (up/down or side to side). If they get into, or accumulate, in the semicircular canals they can cause a sensation of spinning when you lie down or change position. This is not a cause of migraine, but can be a stressor and increase your probability of having a migraine. In other patients, the dizziness comes from other mechanisms in the brain and brainstem.

to as persistent posturo-perceptual dizziness (PPPD) in some medical literature. In vestibular migraine patients, this type of chronic recurrent dizziness symptoms, not vertigo, are predominant (Vuralli, 2017).

This type of dysfunction is not with the vestibular sensors, but the areas in the brain and brainstem to which those sensors project. These areas also take in visual and proprioceptive information in order to give the brain the most accurate perception possible of where you are in space. In order to evaluate this, we look at eye function, balance, posture, and gait patterns, etc. to make sure that these areas are not causing undue stress on the system. This happens when one or two of these systems do not agree. For example, if your vestibular system says that you are falling backward, but your eyes and neck muscles say that you are not, your brain has to decide which sensory systems to trust and which to ignore. Short term this can cause dizziness or disorientation, but long term it can cause a feeling of fogginess or just not feeling very steady. The default of the brain when this happens is to tighten up the neck and back muscles in order to protect itself. After all, if you don't know exactly where you are, your brain will always choose safety over function and lock things down. You can imagine that if this discrepancy causes tight muscles or aberrant eye movements or disorientation, those stressors can all lead to a higher probability of having a migraine.

After treating hundreds, if not over a thousand, migraine patients, I can tell you that almost every one has some type of oculomotor or vestibular dysfunction. Sometimes it's overt and easy to spot and sometimes it's subtle, but rarely is it absent. I've seen multiple patients that had a profound difficulty simply following a target with their eyes, such as me moving my finger in front of them. Rehabbing just the way their eyes moved up and down improved their headaches almost immediately. I had one patient where we simply did eye/head rehabilitation and got rid of a chronic daily two-year migraine in three days! While this isn't the typical home run type of case I expect, when I first saw this type of aberrancy in the patient's examination I knew it was the primary contributor to the headaches.

CHAPTER 8

NEUROLOGICAL DYSFUNCTION

The debate over the cause of migraine, mainly between the vascular and neural theories, has been going on for centuries. Approximately 150 years ago the British physician Edward Liveing (1832–1919) describes migraine as the result of "nerve-storm, discharge of nerve force, or neurosal seizure" (Liveing, 1873). That same year, professor Peter Wallwork (1832–1923) claimed that migraine was due to vascular mechanisms, mainly by vasodilation (Latham, 1873). The vascular theory has been popular over the years, simply saying that the pain associated with migraine is due to the blood vessels in the brain enlarging and putting pressure on the dura and nociceptors (pain receptors). This is actually how I was initially taught to think about migraine, and did for quite some time, because conceptually I could wrap my head around it. The idea that these blood vessels were putting undue pressure on certain areas of the brain and causing pain, in addition to the pulsatile nature of migraine, never led me to question or think any different. When I was first learning about functional neurology, migraine was presented as a primarily neurological dysfunction. This opened me up to the possibility that something more was going on.

ION CHANNEL DYSFUNCTION

At the cellular level, the mechanisms that actually lead to the 'fatiguing' or 'failing' nature of neuronal pools is due to changes in various ion channels. Ion channels help to maintain the cells resting membrane potential. Cells must have a net negative charge in order to have the ability to depolarize and produce an action potential (i.e. a nerve impulse). If there are disruptions in the ability to keep certain ions in or out, then this charge can climb closer to threshold and take less activation in order to fire off. Most studies observe a lowered threshold for neuronal activation in migraine patients compared with controls, which suggest that migraine may result from an altered state of neuronal excitability (Yan, 2014).

There are many types of ion channels that have been implicated in the pathophysiology of migraine, including ASICs, TRPs, P2X, and TRESK (Yan, 2014). There have been many attempts to use this information to create drugs that would selectively target these ion channels, but none have been very successful to date. I believe that the reason this is true is due to the fact that no single ion channel causes migraine, the same way no single gene causes migraine. Since disruption to any ion channel has the potential to shift the resting membrane potential and lead to altered neuronal excitability, migraine can be 'caused' by disruptions to any of the

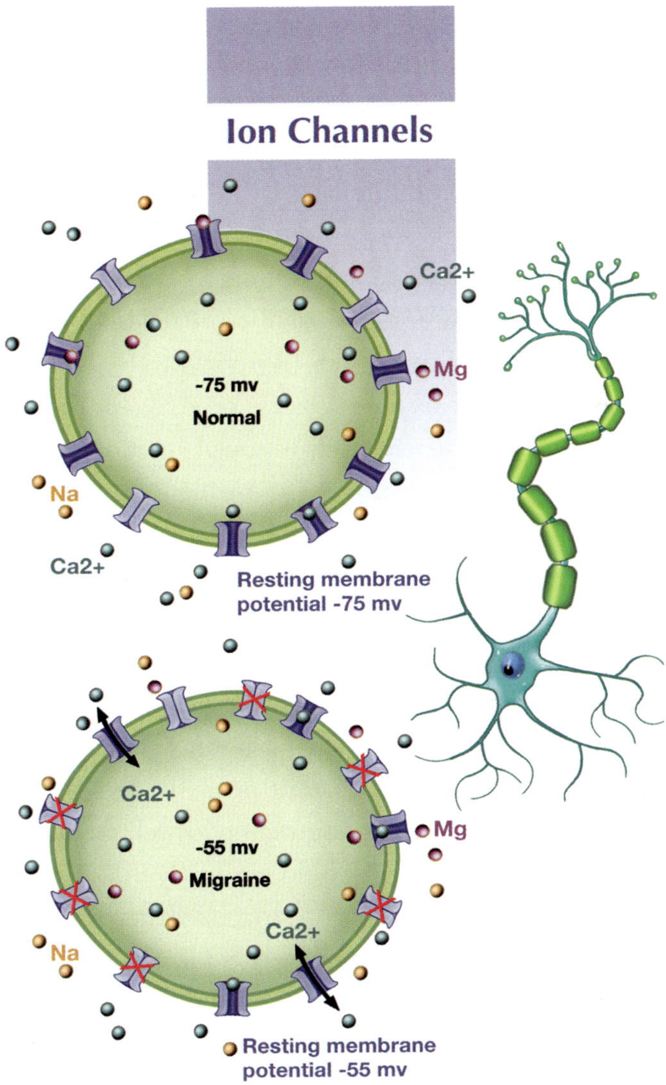

A normal cell with intact ion channels should maintain a resting membrane potential of approximately –75 mv. This means that the inside of the cell is at a more negative charge than outside of the cell membrane. In migraine patients, there are ion channel disruptions that cause an alteration of the resting membrane potential, bringing it closer to threshold and more likely to fire (hyper-excitable). There are many different genes and ion channels implicated in migraine, but the commonality is that it causes an alteration in this resting membrane potential.

channels. The focus should be on how to restore normal neuronal excitability, not on individual ion channels. This is a classic 'can't see the forest for the trees' scenario in which we've zoomed in too far looking for pathophysiology, missing the overall outcome of individual ion channel dysfunction.

Where I start to take a leap clinically is using this information of altered neuronal excitability and linking it with the understanding that protein expression is a dynamic process that can be rapidly induced by extracellular signals (Aymoz, 2016). Knowing that stimulation of neurons can produce new proteins for the cell (such as those that support ion channels and cell membrane integrity) leads to the idea that activation of those neurons will influence the resting membrane potential of those cells. If we can identify and isolate the areas of the brain that have this altered neuronal excitability, then stimulate them in a way that leads to protein production (but not so much that it overwhelms the cells and leads to migraine) we would expect a change in migraine presentation. Conceptually, if a cell was at a resting potential of -58 millivolts (mV), and you are able to stimulate it properly over time, the increase in protein production, strengthening of cell membrane, and repair of damaged ion channels could gradually improve it to -59, -60, all the way to -65 or -70 mV. Obviously this is a conceptual construct, as I am unable to measure these levels during exam or treatment.

This is the basic premise that I have been using over the last few years to develop and modify our treatment modalities. It is also why I believe that no two migraine patients can be treated the same way. Not only would you need to stimulate the correct area of the brain, you would also need to do it in an amount that is intense enough to make a change, but not so intense that it leads to a migraine. I've seen many patients that tried therapies that were actually good for them, but because it was 'too much of a good thing', the therapy led to a migraine so now they avoid it at all costs. This could be an exercise, treatment, or even lifestyle change. This concept is why we talk about the 'bucket getting bigger' as treatment continues. If your resting membrane potential is getting more stable, your bucket is getting bigger and you can compensate for more and more stressors on the body.

Patient Story

Susan

Susan was one of our first hemiplegic migraine cases. She was the quintessential 'doing everything right' patient. She had the cleanest diet I had ever seen, worked out intensely, but without overtraining, and had a positive demeanor. Due to all of these factors, she was only experiencing hemiplegic episodes every two or three months. However, she reported that they were becoming more frequent over time.

Susan's lab tests showed an odd pattern for her circadian rhythm, indicative of parasitic infection. We ran a gastrointestinal (GI) test and found that she had a minor GI infection that wasn't causing any stomach problems, but was causing chronic low-level inflammation. We treated both the hormonal dysfunction and parasite while performing neurological rehabilitation. We have been able to follow her over four or five years and found that she has only had one or two recurrence of her symptoms, always following an extremely stressful and/or exhausting period of time.

Had she not had such a stellar diet and lifestyle patterns, there is a good chance that her symptoms would have progressed significantly before we had ever seen her. She is now able to recognize exactly how much stress/poor diet/lack of sleep/alcohol/etc. it takes in combination to cause an attack. Many times she will have a number of these things occur all at once and she will still not have an episode. The ability to understand migraine and take control of it – instead of it taking control of you – is the most important aspect of everything that we do during my program with patients.

AUTONOMIC DYSFUNCTION

It wasn't until I started seeing neurological differences in migraine patients of my own that I began to explore the idea that the condition may be more brain-based, and therefore treatment should be focused on brain mechanisms and not vascular ones. Autonomic dysfunction has been identified as a component of migraine for quite some time, but has been controversial as to how it is dysfunctional. One area that I think is vital for future advancements in migraine treatment is the understanding of how the autonomic nervous system can become dysfunctional in people who suffer from the condition, and what testing is most reliable when developing a diagnosis. A simple, easy to administer autonomic nervous system (ANS) testing mechanism would help us better identify true migraine versus other headache disorders that often get confused with migraine.

As described in chapter two, the first consistent finding I began to see in migraine patients was that they tend to have a difference in blood pressure (BP) from side to side. Research has suggested for years that primary care physicians should take bilateral blood pressure (Martin, 2013; Grossman, 2013; Cassidy, 2001). However, of those physicians that are aware of this (77%), only 30% agreed with the recommendation (Martin, 2013). In a busy practice, it can be difficult to properly measure bilateral blood pressure, let alone retake it if the results are concerning. Therefore very few of our patients have ever had their blood pressure taken in this manner.

There are different ways to take bilateral blood pressure, but we prefer to do it simultaneously with automatic brachial cuffs. This is a more reliable method and should be preferred over sequential blood pressure assessment as it is less influenced by extraneous effects (van der Hoeven, 2013; Fotherby, 1993). This type of blood pressure technique has also been shown to be reproducible between visits, indicating that if we see a difference at re-examination, the change is likely due to treatment. This technique also shows no age-related differences (Fotherby, 1993).

If you read through the papers referenced on this topic in addition to many others, you'll see that there really is no consensus as to 'normal' differences in BP from side to side. Some papers say that it is higher on the right or left, and some say there is no difference whatsoever. Initially, this was thought to be due to the use of traditional sphygmomanometers, which are subject to user error and differences in interpretation. Currently, I believe it is due to the many different devices and methods in which the blood pressure is taken. Based on these facts, it is my opinion that in a clinical setting the most reliable way to use this information is to apply the exact same methods and environment to take a BP reading in your own office. Then you can use your findings over time to see if your healthy population has increased or decreased BP on one side versus the other consistently.

In or our office, we typically see that if you take bilateral BP, the left side will be two to three points higher (systolic) than the right side in healthy, non-migrainous patients. This is thought to be due to the fact that the aorta goes to the left and therefore will naturally have increased pressure. So if someone has a BP eight points higher on the left or three points higher on the right, I would consider them equally as significant. In Western medicine, you wouldn't get too concerned about BP differences from side to side unless they were more than 20 mmHg, which can indicate peripheral arterial disease (Mehlsen, 2014). However, that is looking at the cardiovascular consequences of BP and not the neurological ones.

If your BP is high, say 145/90, there are obvious cardiovascular risks and concerns associated with those findings. You would still expect that the opposite side is similar to that reading, so 145/90 on the left, 142/90 on the right would be considered normal. If you have 145/90 on the left, there is no reason why your BP should be 150/90 on the right. While this wouldn't pose any more of a cardiovascular risk, it raises the question, 'why isn't the nervous system controlling both sides equally?' This finding by itself doesn't confirm a migraine diagnosis, but it begins to make the case that there is a difference from one side to the other that could be attributed to the pathophysiology of migraine.

As discussed in chapter 2, this difference in the two sides points to an imbalance in the autonomic nervous system (ANS). You can think of the autonomic nervous system as simply a way to get fuel to the correct area of the body at the correct time. It is broken into two main divisions: the sympathetic and the parasympathetic nervous systems. The sympathetic system is the one typically known as the 'fight or flight' response. So if a tiger jumps out in front of you, you want all the fuel you can get to your muscles in order to run away as fast as possible. The other side, the parasympathetic system, is called the 'rest and digest' or 'feed and breed' system. This system is active when you are trying to digest food, repair damaged tissue, heal from an illness, or prepare for sexual activity. So while these two systems seem to be at odds, they are just two parts of the same system that get blood to the right areas at the right time.

The control of this system starts in the brain. There are multiple areas in the cortex that contribute to autonomic function, but the hypothalamus is usually the area thought of as the starting point for activation of the ANS. While the hypothalamus controls global autonomic function, there are areas in the brainstem and spinal cord that help control ANS function on each side of the body. For example, if you were using your right arm to throw a ball, you wouldn't want to activate the sympathetic system globally and send blood to every muscle, only the ones helping the right arm to throw the ball. So while the hypothalamus allows for global activation of the autonomic nervous system, areas in your brainstem and spinal cord regulate the activity from side to side. This allows for proper fuel delivery to only the area that needs it. In patients where this mechanism fails, you'll see that they have 'sympathetic escape' where they will become flush, have discoloration of their hands or feet, begin sweating, or even feel anxious. These are all examples of improper control of the autonomic nervous system.

As I described in chapter 2, the research is back and forth between what type of autonomic dysfunction is occurring in migraine. One paper describes an increase in functional connectivity between the hypothalamus and those brain regions involved in regulation of autonomic functions, including the locus coeruleus, caudate, parahippocampal gyrus, cerebellum, and temporal pole (Moulton, 2014). The author makes the argument that this functional connectivity could globally alter autonomic function, not specifically the sympathetic or parasympathetic division.

The reason I believe that there is this disparity in findings is due to the fact that the ANS is controlled at different segmental levels in the brainstem, such as the periaqueductal gray, parabrachial nucleus, ventrolateral medulla, dorsal motor vagal nucleus, and the nucleus of the solitary tract (Schwartz, 2013). These areas are either directly involved with migraine or are part of what's known as the 'reticular formation' that is closely associated with the areas involved with an attack. So if patient A has more dysfunction in their upper right brainstem, their treatment would be markedly different to that of patient B with more dysfunction in the lower left brainstem. If you can then find different exercises or therapies that stimulate that area of the brainstem, you can strengthen it like a muscle. For example, horizontal eye movements are controlled primarily in the pons and medulla (lower brainstem), while vertical eye movements are controlled in the mesencephalon and pons (upper brainstem). In the patient that has more dysfunction in the lower brainstem, they will do better with horizontal eye movements

Autonomic Asymmetry of the Nervous System

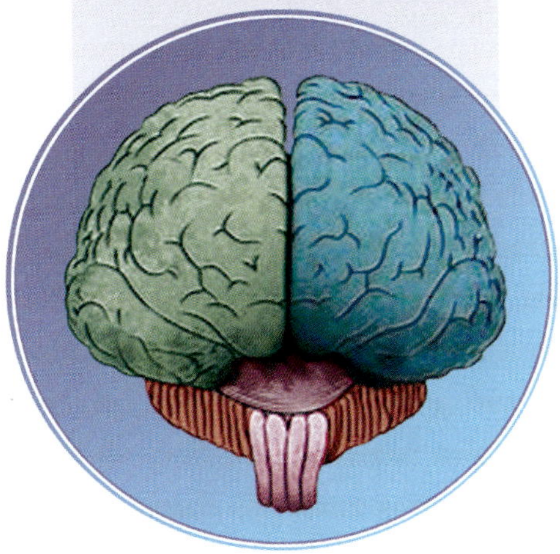

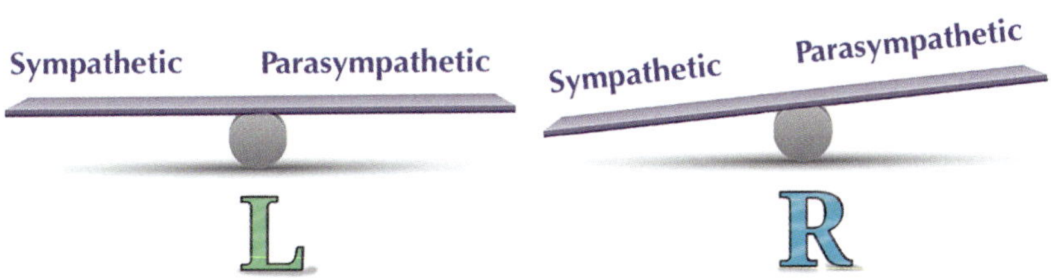

When any part of the autonomic regulatory system is dysfunctional, there can be an imbalance between the two parts (sympathetic and parasympathetic). This imbalance is commonly found in migraine patients and is often times very subtle. Examining things like blood pressure on each side or oxygen saturation on each side can give a window into this possible imbalance.

as therapy as opposed to the patient that has more dysfunction in the upper brainstem. These exercises can then strengthen areas in the brainstem that are found to be aberrant in migraine so they become healthier and are less likely to fail and lead to a migraine. This allows us to target our therapy so that a similar treatment for patient A can be modified in a way to make it more beneficial for patient B. Some of the techniques we are using to address these issues already have great research on their efficacy, but some are experimental. We are currently working on a few research studies for the techniques that have not been researched yet.

Patient Story

Jessica

Jessica was experiencing migraines and headaches every day and had been for two years before coming to see us. She lived out of state but had recently had to move back home with her parents due to the debilitating nature of the headaches. She was unable to work and had not experienced relief with any previous mode of treatment.

Her neurological examination was relatively good, with a main finding of autonomic dysfunction. However, her hormonal testing showed significant dysfunction with her response to stress. She was also found to have neurogenic inflammation of the C2 nerve root in the cervical vertebrae, which was contributing to the headache she experienced in the back of her head.

After a week of intensive treatment, we followed up with Jessica for the next few weeks. She was able to keep her headache below a 1/10 on the pain scale for the next month! Unfortunately, she got a pretty severe sinus infection that spiked her headaches back up for one or two weeks. When the infection was dealt with, she went back down to a 0–1/10 headache every day. She was able to move back home and resume a normal life. We caught up with her a year later to find that she continued to do well and even decided to travel abroad for the next year.

OTHER NEUROLOGICAL CONTRIBUTIONS

Another interesting aspect of eye movements is that they share some of the same parts of the brain and are functionally connected through what is known as 'homologous columns'. Homologous columns are areas of the brain that develop together and maintain functional connections, but migrate to different areas of the brain. For example, the cranial nerves 3, 4, 6, and 12 are in the same homologous column (Schwarts, 2013). The first three cranial nerves (3, 4, and 6) control the eyes and the 12th cranial nerve controls tongue movement. These connections can be helpful when attempting to stimulate a part of the brain that is unstable and cannot be directly targeted. So if I wanted to stimulate the eyes to help keep them steady, but they are fatiguing very quickly, I can have the patient do various tongue exercises to steady them. Admittedly the first time I heard about this type of application it sounded crazy, but after seeing hundreds of patients in this manner, the outcomes are surprisingly consistent and predictable.

Just for reference, here are the main areas involved with processing and modulating the trigeminal pain pathways related to migraine:

Superior salivatory nucleus
Rostral ventromedial medulla (RVM)
Nucleus raphe magnus (NRM)
Parabrachial nucleus
Locus coeruleus
Ventrolateral periaqueductal gray (vl-PAG)
Cuneiform nucleus
Hypothalamic nuclei (anterior, lateral, posterior, ventromedial, perifornical, supraoptic)

Thalamus (VPM, posterior, intralaminar)
(Goadsby, 2017)

As you can see, these areas include all parts of the brainstem (medulla, pons, and mesencephalon) in addition to many areas of the hypothalamus and thalamus. There are also studies that indicate that the cerebral cortex – mainly the insular and somatosensory cortices – are also involved in modulating the pain response associated with migraine. Patients with greater symptoms of allodynia, for example, have been shown to have smaller midbrain volumes. Patients with lower heat pain thresholds have smaller medullary and cerebellar volumes (Chong, 2016). In the cortex, voxel-based morphometric studies show significant reductions in the middle frontal and inferior frontal cortex in migraine patients, possibly accounting for cognitive, emotional, or autonomic dysfunction (Hu, 2015). These areas would show up as 'normal' when looking at magnetic resonance imaging (MRI) as brain volume decreases are typically only noted if they are significantly or pathologically diminished.

So if you apply the understanding that all of these areas have the ability to be involved in migraine, but are not all involved with every patient, you can begin to understand why there is a wide disparity in research findings. If someone has migraine mainly due to cortical dysfunction and they are treated with brainstem modulators, the outcome might not be so great. This is why customized care must be applied to each individual migraine patient.

Another interesting concept is the global cortical involvement of the left and right hemispheres of the brain relating to migraine. The left hemisphere affects predominantly parasympathetic function while the right hemisphere affects primarily sympathetic function. By comparing patients that had primarily left- or right-sided migraine, they found that left-sided migraine patients had higher forehead vasodilatation and bradycardia (an abnormally slow heart rate) in response to ocular irritation, indicating higher somatoparasympathetic responsiveness (Avnon, 2004). Targeting the left or right hemisphere based on the type of autonomic dysfunction could be another avenue of investigation relating to treatment of migraine, but it has not been explored as of yet.

While this may seem like a lot of effort, the outcome and savings over the long run would be astronomical on a national and global level. You would see a decrease in pharmaceutical costs, diminished amounts of lost wages due to time being taken off work, decreased visits to the doctor, and increased amounts of productivity due to patients not needing to constantly recover.

SPECTRUM OF MIGRAINE

An important concept in the overall understanding of the condition is the spectrum of migraine dysfunction. On one end there are the patients that have a migraine all day everyday. On the other there are the patients that get one migraine every couple of years. If you are susceptible to migraine, you are *always* susceptible to migraine, but that doesn't mean you have to have them all the time. In order to be on the far end of the spectrum, the person must have a very small bucket. If their bucket is in an area of the brainstem that does not get much natural stimulation, the bucket will get smaller over time due to lack of activation. This also occurs if the bucket is in an area that tends to flair up during migraine attacks, such as the midbrain, and is therefore voided by the patient. For example, if the patient's main dysfunction is in the midbrain, they may avoid light and sound because it triggers a migraine. If you understand the bucket theory, you can understand why the key is not to avoid those type of activities, but find the level of stimulation that the patient can handle without overstimulating them and leading to a migraine. This will strengthen the area of the brain and basically make the bucket bigger, leading to the patient becoming more and more resistant to migraine attacks over time. (Image #4 - Migraine Scale)

I believe this concept is why many practitioners tell me they hate treating migraine. They'll say that they treat one person with a certain therapy and it's a miracle, but the next patient responds terribly. They may be doing the perfect treatment for that patient, but it's just too much of a good thing. They also may only be addressing one of the two or three aspects that are leading to migraines. If we can help the patient understand the concept of being on the spectrum of migraine and the bucket theory, they can help control many of the 'bucket fillers' and largely manage their migraines on their own after proper treatment. It will also help to explain why attacks are beginning to increase after a time when they have been having very few migraines. Keeping on track with properly prescribed brain exercises, dietary adherence, stress reduction, hormonal regulation, and general healthy practices will continue to move the patient down the spectrum toward less and less migraine.

Ever since I began using this analogy to explain migraine, nearly every person I talk with grasps the concept and expresses how simple it really is to understand. Another way to explain the long-term outcome is to compare it to physical exercise. Imagine that you go the gym to work on your core muscles because your back hurts and you feel weak. You workout five times a week for four months and not only feel better, you also have a six pack now! If you were to then stop working out and not eat right, it would seem rather odd to complain to your personal trainer a year down the road that their training method 'didn't continue to work'. That's just not how the body works. If you have dysfunction in certain parts of the brain that make you susceptible to migraine and you work really hard to improve it, not maintaining that improvement will likely lead to more migraines. This is why I try to keep in contact with all of my migraine patients on some type of regular basis. It doesn't have to be that often, just enough to check in, ask about habits, diet, exercise, etc., and if anything is getting too far off track we can nip it in the bud before it starts to cause a backslide. In the same way your six pack takes much less effort to maintain once it's achieved, but would require a lot more effort it you let your body go back to where you started.

BRAIN STATE THEORY

There are a few reasons I waited to write this book until now, the main one being that I had this concept of how migraine worked in my mind and from what I had seen from my patients, but I didn't yet have a comprehensive way to express it through research. The research was all there in many different pieces, but there was no comprehensive model that gave direct credibility to what I was seeing. Luckily, a great paper came out in 2017 that gave one of the most comprehensive reviews of migraine pathology that I had ever seen. The most exciting part was the final conclusion that migraine was an altered brain state at the root of everything. The paper summed up their findings as follows:

> "An alternative and all-encompassing hypothesis is that the brain is at the heart of triggering migraine. Rather than a sequential activation of different brain regions, migraine is a disorder of the brain and therefore considered a 'brain state', and is a consequence of changes, or dysfunction, in brainstem and hypothalamic regions, which contribute to changes in cellular and vascular function in many regions of the brain."
>
> (Goadsby, 2017)

The authors summed up their findings of more than 900 research papers into a concise understanding of what was happening.

What we see in our office is that this altered brain state is an alteration in the central integrated state (CIS) of a pool of neurons. The central integrated state is simply the overall health of a neuron. Normally, a neuron has what's called a 'resting membrane potential' of about -65 mV (Schwartz, 2013). This means that the neuron has a negative charge inside of the cell. In order to 'fire' or send a signal, the neuron must reach a threshold of about -55 mV, which then initiates an action potential that allows the neuron to send signals to other cells. If a cell is not healthy and not producing enough proteins and energy to maintain its -65 mV level, it will slowly start to creep closer and closer to the -55 mV potential. This means that it takes less and less stimulation in order for it to fire off. It also means that it has less of an ability to maintain its firing potential and therefore fatigues more quickly.

If this occurs to the areas that are affected by migraine, it becomes easier and easier to have a migraine. Many more stimuli become triggers, and the headaches become more frequent, more intense, and last longer. If you fail to identify and stimulate the correct areas of the brain, this spiral unfortunately continues. I have heard the same story over and over to the point where it's almost unbelievable how much and how long people have suffered with this continually worsening condition.

If you apply this principle to migraine, you can begin to understand why stimulation of certain neurons associated with migraine could make those areas healthier and less likely to fatigue. While many other areas are involved in modulating pain, ultimately the trigeminal nucleus is responsible for the agony associated with migraine. If this area is unhealthy, it doesn't take much stimulation at all in order for it to fire, and therefore send signals to the brain that cause the perception of intense pain. If you are able to stimulate this area, and other areas involved with modulating this process, you can bring their resting membrane potential further and further away from -55 mV, making the patient less and less likely to have migraines. The reason that stimulation of the trigeminal nucleus itself doesn't lead to total resolution of pain is due to the fact that so many other areas help modulate it. These areas can also be affected from an altered 'brain state' and therefore must be stimulated as well. If you only stimulate the trigeminal area the results will generally be better than doing nothing, but will not be consistent or complete. We hear that more and more patients are trying this method due to improvements in research and product development. It's great that these methods are being brought to light, but caution must be used in hailing any one treatment as the 'be-all and end-all'.

I've found when speaking with other healthcare professionals that the idea of the Central Integrated State (CIS) of a neuron is somewhat foreign and difficult to conceptualize. In traditional medicine, for example, the body is generally thought to either be healthy or not healthy. You either have a tumor or you don't, diabetes or normal blood sugar, hypertension or not. While there are some gray areas, generally if the x-rays, MRIs, CTs, and blood work, etc. all look clean, then there must not be anything wrong. As I just described, the neuron can be functional and not show any problem on imaging, but can be getting closer to threshold and ultimately unhealthier.

Think of it this way: imagine you have two 80-year-old men that want to run a marathon. They both have no overt diseases, they can walk, run, breath normally, etc. However, the first 80-year-old currently runs 10 miles a day and the other one hasn't run more than a block in 20 years. If you have both of them start training by running 10 miles, what do you think will happen? It's not that the second person can't run 10 miles eventually, but his current fitness level will limit his ability to perform. There's nothing 'wrong' with him, but he is functionally not as healthy as the first person.

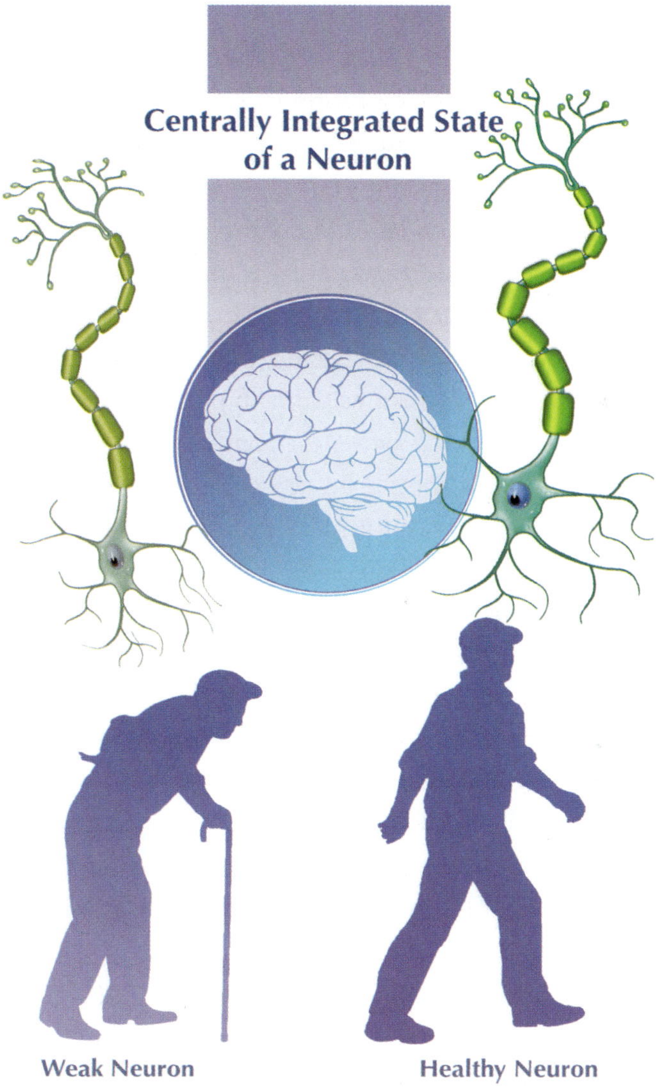

The centrally integrated state (CIS) of a neuron is essentially how healthy it is. Neurons are not just dead or alive, they have a spectrum of health and function. Think of it like this, if you take two eighty year old men and compare their running ability, you wouldn't just see if they could run or not. You would test to see how far they could run and how long it takes them to do so. If the first man can run ten miles and the second one can only run a quarter mile, they are both performing the same task but are obviously at different health and functional levels. The same goes for neurons.

In migraine patients, the genetic predisposition essentially makes certain pools of neurons like the second guy – nothing technically 'wrong' with those neurons, but it's not as functionally healthy as the neurons in someone who does not have the predisposition for migraine.

This new concept of migraine pathology, specifically relating to the CIS of various neuronal pools, is one that needs further research. Now that the idea of an altered brain state exists, the next hurdle is to show that in each specific migraineur there is dysfunction in specific areas. If we can use some type of imaging or quantifiable measurement for each patient, treatment options will be more specific and outcomes should be more predictable. This will also allow practitioners to have a simple, easy to understand applications for any brain region that is involved. Until this is available, physical examination will remain the gold standard in diagnosing these functional deficiencies.

CHAPTER 9

GENETICS

Genetics play an obvious and inherent role in the pathophysiology of migraine. Many studies have aimed at identifying the specific gene that causes the condition and have made some progress, but have not nailed down one factor. In reality, many different genetic variations have been associated with migraine. For example, dopamine receptor D2 (DRD2) has been significantly associated with risk of migraine in female patients (Deng, 2018). Familial hemiplegic migraine (FHM) has been associated with a number of mutations. FHM1 is caused by mutations in the CACNA1A gene, FHM2 is caused by mutations in the ATP1A2 gene, and FHM3 is caused by mutations in the SCN1A gene (Schwarz, 2018; Dhifallah, 2018). A study in China suggested that brain-derived neurotrophic factor (BDNF) rs6265 and rs2049046 polymorphism were associated with common migraine (Cai, 2018). There are a number of others, but I think you get the point.

Family history can also influence how migraine impacts a person. Migraine frequency, for example, has been shown to be increased in males only with a family history of migraine. A stronger family history of migraine is also associated with a lower age-at-onset, higher number of medication days, and migraine with aura (Pelzer, 2018). An aura is most commonly visual, but it can include other symptoms such as sensory disturbances, speech difficulty, facial drooping, and numbness/tingling etc.

There has also been recent research showing that specific genetic alterations lead to certain foods triggering or impacting migraine patients (De Marchis, 2018). This means that not every migraine patients needs to stay away from chocolate or wine, but you wouldn't know unless you tested for the genetic variations.

I believe that the reason many different genes are associated with migraine is the same reason that many different areas of the brain are associated with the condition. This disorder is an altered brain state, and specific genetic alterations will cause certain types of increased stress in the system, making you more likely to have migraine. Think of it in terms of the bucket theory, if someone has five different genetic variations that are causing stressors that fill up the bucket, they are more likely to have chronic or frequent migraine when compared to the person with one or two genetic variations. If you are filling up a bucket with water hoses, is it going to fill up quicker with one or two hoses or five?

HEMIPLEGIC MIGRAINE

One of the most genetically studied forms of this condition is that of hemiplegic migraine. As discussed earlier in this chapter, there are a few different gene mutations responsible for FHM. This is a type of migraine that can mimic stroke-like symptoms, but has a migrainous etiology. If we again think of the many different areas of the brain that can be affected by migraine, if they were all to fail or fatigue at the same time, it would cause a multitude of symptoms. In my experience, hemiplegic migraines often start out with minor symptoms, such as tingling in the hands, minor facial drooping, visual disturbances, or weakness. As they progress, the symptoms become more pronounced and will occur at the same time. A progressed presentation would involve facial paralysis on one side, as if they were having an actual stroke, difficulty with speech, numbness/tingling down the entire arm/leg, weakness of the entire arm/leg, loss of consciousness, nausea, and fatigue. These attacks can be transient, only lasting a few minutes to an hour, or chronic when they can last for months at a time.

As you can imagine, the first time a hemiplegic migraine occurs the patient will normally go to the emergency room as they are concerned they are having a stroke. This is the correct course of care and should always be considered with these type of symptoms. Once stroke or other neurological pathologies are ruled out, the diagnosis of hemiplegic migraine may be explored. While it's never a bad idea to go back to the emergency room when these episodes occur, most patients will recognize when an episode is coming on and just rest or lie down in a dark room until it has passed. Unfortunately, for some people the episode persists for many months. I have seen patients that are unable to function at all and have episodes that have lasted for over six months! Needless to say this is incredibly debilitating and restricts them from performing normal daily activities.

The fact that they are genetically influenced does not mean that there is nothing that can be done. In fact, hemiplegic migraine is one of my favorite types of migraine to treat due to the speed of response to treatment. With hemiplegia, the key is identifying all of the areas in the brain that have been affected by the migrainous brain state and stimulating them all at the same time. We tend to see that you can push these patients more than normal migraine patients because they will show obvious signs of fatigue when undergoing treatment. This means that the second we see any type of facial drooping or reported symptoms, we stop treatment and allow them to rest. After a few hours we can resume treatment and push them a little further than we did in the previous session. We can then give them simple strategies and exercises that will continue to strengthen the affected areas of the brain and brainstem. Typically patients will continue them for a few weeks after they are feeling better, but will only resume them if the episodes becoming more frequent again.

Patient Story

Elizabeth

Elizabeth contacted us while she was in the middle of a seven-month episode of hemiplegic migraine. They were so severe that she was barely able to get off of the couch for that entire time. When it first occurred, she was experiencing numbness and tingling of her arm and leg, slurred speech, and facial drooping. As you can imagine, this was terrifying and she and her husband rushed to the hospital. She was initially diagnosed as having a stroke, but the imaging didn't reveal any type of cerebrovascular accident (CVA). She was monitored for a bit, but was then released without any suggestions for care.

Through her own research, Elizabeth realized that she may actually be suffering from a hemiplegic migraine and not a stroke. We were able to chat on the phone for a bit and that's what it sounded like to me too. We started her with some dietary changes and hormonal suggestions. Within a month her symptoms had resolved by over 80%! When she came to see us, she was so happy that she was feeling better that she downplayed the other symptoms she was still experiencing. She had some odd indicators regarding her sense of smell in addition to significant balance issues (she was only in her mid 20s). Her balance test results actually showed that her stability was only better than 5% of people her age.

Her examination revealed significant functional deficits of the left hemisphere of the brain and the right lower brainstem. We gave her targeted exercises for these areas, which she will tell you look kind of ridiculous. By the end of the week she reported feeling better than even before she had ever experienced any symptoms.

> When we followed up with her five months later, she reported that she had not had one episode or symptoms since her visit.

EPIGENETICS: IT'S NOT ALL ABOUT THE GENES

The reason we're able to treat things like hemiplegic migraine, or any migraine that have genetic underpinnings for that matter, is due to epigenetics and neural plasticity. Epigenetics comprise both DNA methylation and post-translational modifications of the tails of histone proteins, affecting chromatin structure and gene expression (Eising, 2013). While there is clearly a genetic component to migraine, environmental factors likely contribute almost equal risk to developing the condition (Wessman, 2007). Eising goes on to state that environmental factors may directly trigger migraine attacks or lower the attack threshold by rendering the brain more susceptible to trigger factors. These factors include all of the ones included in this book, as well as hormones, stress, musculoskeletal dysfunction, inflammation, and neurological dysfunction.

Epigenetics can be thought of loosely in terms of building a new house. If you are planning a build you need an architect. The architect will draw up the blueprints to the house so that it can be completed exactly as specified. This is analogous to what a gene does – it has the potential to cause something to happen. However, if those blueprints are never read and implemented by a construction crew, the house doesn't get built. In the same way, if the conditions are not met to 'turn on' or read a gene, there is no gene expression. What the gene actually codes for is known as the genotype, while the actual expression by an organism is known as a phenotype. For

Epigenetics

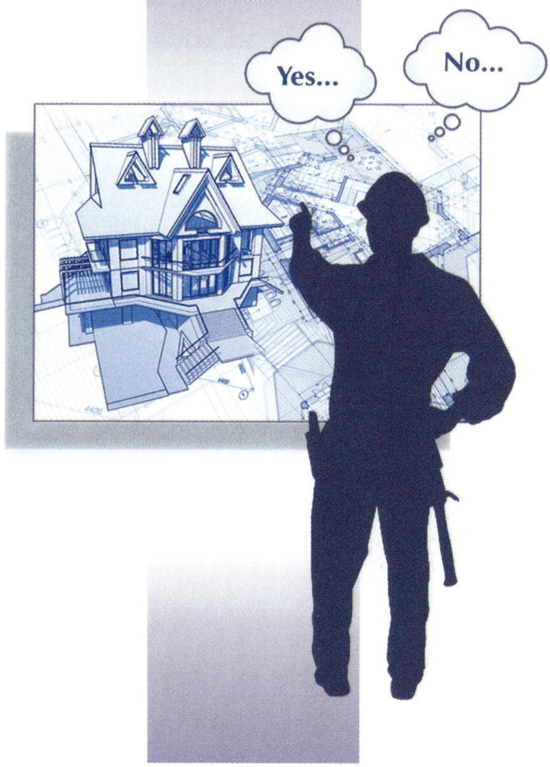

Having a genetic predisposition for something does not guarantee you will express that gene. There are many epigenetic factors that go in to determining which genes are read and which are not. Think of genes like a blueprint to a house. The blueprint itself does not build the house, but rather provides the instructions on how to build it. If the blueprints aren't read, then the house doesn't get built. When a person has the genetic predisposition to migraine, it doesn't mean they have to have migraine all the time, only that they have the blueprints for migraine. By altering their environment (diet, neuro therapies, exercise, etc.) we can help "turn off" certain genes so they are not expressed. This is why we are able to make positive and profound changes in migraine patients, despite their genetic predisposition to the condition.

migraine, the phenotype typically only occurs if the environmental factors allow. This should give a massive amount of hope to anyone who has been long suffering with migraine: a genetic predisposition to migraine does not guarantee that you have to suffer with them forever. By changing environmental factors appropriately and comprehensively, you can massively change the migraine phenotype. This is why we can see drastic reductions in migraine days, intensity, and duration with treatment. This is also why some people respond incredibly well to dietary changes or medication or chiropractic or acupuncture or massage or herbs or Botox or nerve stimulation, while others see no noticeable improvement. If you feel like your case is hopeless and there's nothing you can do, just remember that your blueprints haven't been read properly yet.

CHAPTER 10

NUTRITION

"You have to try _______ diet, it totally got rid of my migraines!" "You have to try ______ product, it totally got rid of my migraines!" If you've experienced migraine for more than two days you've undoubtedly had this happen to you multiple times, all said by well-meaning people. Now there's nothing wrong with suggesting something that has helped you get rid of migraines, why wouldn't you want to help someone else? The frustration begins to set in for chronic migraine sufferers when they've heard the same things over and over again, because they've already tried each and every suggestion, probably twice.

Nutrition is part of migraine just like any other trigger. It plays a huge part with some people and not much with others. So one of the first things I discuss with patients that have already tried nutrition or any type of supplement is the bucket theory. If the only thing filling up your bucket is nutritional stressors, a healthy diet would most likely 'cure' your migraines. Now as we know they're not really cured as a patient is still susceptible, but we took out the main driver of their migraine. For most chronic migraine patients, however, diet is a part of the solution, but not all of it. Many times we will place patients on a diet somewhat similar to what they have done in the past, with the understanding that it's not a cure, but it does stack the deck in our favor. If someone gets significantly better through mainly neurological treatment, but are still having symptoms, their diet may be the part that pushes them over the edge to feeling significantly better. In my opinion, why not start out with that to begin with?

Something else that comes up quite a bit is that some things I generally recommend might be a trigger for migraine or could cause problems. There are two reasons to better understand why this is not the case. First, there has recently been research showing how some of the more common triggers for migraine actually have a genetic component (De Marchis, 2018). So if you suffer migraine and have gene 'x' then chocolate may be a bad food for you. However, if you don't have gene 'x' then it's really not a big deal. This can happen with anything from alcohol to bread to even citrus fruits and nuts. Therefore, we generally cut out many of these foods initially, but slowly re-introduce them one at a time to see what is reactive and what is not. We can also run food sensitivity panels to narrow down what may be a trigger.

Some patients find that they are sensitive to many different foods, which generally leads us to believe that there is some type of intestinal hyperpermeability or leaky gut. This occurs when the tight junctions in the intestine break apart and allow for small particles of food to get through and react with the immune system. Since these particles are entering the body inappropriately, the immune system identifies them as foreign invaders and mounts an immune response to them. This is generally how you find people that are sensitive to seemingly harmless or healthy foods such as carrots or pineapple.

Patient Story

Barbara

Barbara was a 25-year-old woman with a 13-year history of migraine. She was having five migraines a week when she came to see us. She had tried everything from diet changes to acupuncture to Botox, but nothing seemed to help.

When we started Barbara on a dietary regimen, she noted that she had tried a few diets very similar to this one, but with slight variations. After being on the diet for only a month, she noticed that her migraines had already been cut in half! For this particular patient, the blood sugar regulatory aspect of the diet was a huge contributor to her migraines. Once the blood sugar was under control, her headaches began to be under control.

During her week with us, we saw a pretty strong pattern of right-sided lower brainstem dysfunction. Barbara noticed that on the second day she felt like she was going to get a migraine, but it never manifested. This is one of the most common signs we see that indicate the migraines are beginning to regress. We were able to keep her migraine to one attack during the week that also coincided with the beginning of her cycle.

After our one-week intensive treatment program where we see people three or four times a day to make the greatest change in the shortest amount of time, Barbara did have a one-day migraine attack, which is unusual, but it also woke her in the middle of the night. After that, she had one or two migraines in the subsequent month and has continued to improve since then. She had many different factors contributing to her condition, but addressing them all at once allowed her to get off of the medication and reduce her migraines by over 90%.

CAFFEINE

Another big component to nutrition is caffeine. I know I'm going to lose a few of you with this, but bear with me. Caffeine is a drug. It is the most widely consumed drug on the planet, but it's still a drug, meaning that it should only be used when necessary. Most people think of caffeine in conjunction with coffee, but it is present in tea, soda, energy drinks, and chocolate, etc. Also, even decaf coffee has a percentage of caffeine in it, so that won't work as a substitute. With migraine, it's used in many medications because it can help with the pain during an attack, just like Triptans or other abortive medications. However, caffeine is not a treatment – in fact it tends to make things worse. One study even showed that stopping caffeine helped with how well medications worked on migraine when patients were having an acute attack (Lee, 2016). We know that when used specifically for the acute attacks of migraine, adding caffeine with the abortive medication used helps reduce symptoms better than using either one by itself (Lipton, 2017).

This leads to my basic tenant of caffeine and migraine: use it like you would use Triptans or any abortive medications – only when you need it. If you are on daily amounts of caffeine, you are more likely to progress from episodic to chronic migraine (Scher, 2004). When caffeine is used on a regular basis we develop a tolerance to it, meaning that without it we will have withdrawal symptoms. If you are already having migraines on a frequent basis, the increase in headaches from missing a day or two of coffee is enough to make you throw up your hands and swear that you'll never stop drinking it. Many of my patients report that they've tried to stop ingesting caffeine, but when they do they feel terrible and have to go back on it. This is due to the fact that caffeine withdrawal follows a common 'bell curve' of symptoms.

After helping hundreds of people give up caffeine, here is the typical progression. The first day will not be too bad as the body hasn't really noticed the change. You may be somewhat fatigued, but that's about it. The second and third day are usually the worst, with headache, fatigue, and mood changes being very common. Typically by the fourth or fifth day your body has started to adjust and you are feeling much better. Based on this pattern, I've come up with a simple protocol for cutting out caffeine.

You can go cold turkey or drink less and less if you feel more comfortable that way. If you are drinking more than two cups of caffeine per day, I would recommend gradually reducing your intake before you come off it completely. If you work a normal Monday–Friday, have your last cup of caffeine on Thursday. This way, Friday isn't so bad, you can rest/recover/sleep etc. during Saturday and Sunday, and by Monday or Tuesday you're feeling pretty good. You'll notice that instead of morning energy from tea or coffee, followed by a crash in the afternoon, you'll have a nice consistent level of energy after getting off caffeine. I've had people try to do this by starting on Monday and it ruins their whole week.

For those of you that think you can't do it, I'll tell you about the meanest look I ever got from a patient. I had a young lady that was having migraines almost daily come in for an initial exam. When we sat down to discuss treatment options, I asked about her caffeine intake and she said she drank coffee. When I asked how much, she replied, "about eight a day". I said, "wow eight cups per day, that's quite a lot – we're going to have to slowly decrease that amount". She said, "No not eight cups – eight pots!" EIGHT POTS! I couldn't believe it. So needless to say, when I told her it's imperative to cut out the caffeine, I saw literal daggers come out of her eyes right at me.

After that discussion, I never saw her again (perhaps not surprisingly). Luckily I was also treating her partner for something else. He told me about two months later that she had actually listened to what I had said and gradually cut down to no coffee after about a month and a half! The greatest part was she stopped having migraines and swore off coffee because of how dramatic the change was to her health! So when someone says that they just couldn't go without their morning coffee, I know it's playing a big part in their overall migraine picture. Caffeine is starting to fill their bucket every morning without them even knowing it.

MASTERING MIGRAINE DIET

As discussed earlier in the chapter, many different factors play into what will be the best diet for any one individual. That's why with each patient we tailor their diet based on any known allergies, triggers, or sensitivities that have been discovered. For some people this creates a very different diet than I normally prescribe, while for others they can stay pretty close to the basic outline of the migraine diet. I will discuss the basic premise of the diet in this chapter, with the caveat that this is not a 'one size fits all' diet and must be customized based on individual differences.

The basic premise for the diet is simple: gluten and dairy-free, no caffeine, no alcohol. There is plenty of discussion about whether or not gluten is inflammatory or bad for everyone, or if a gluten free diet is healthy. What I can tell you is that a gluten-free diet on its own is not healthy. If you are eating gluten-free, but all you eat is gluten-free cookies and pasta and breads and candy, etc., that is not a healthy diet. However, we do know that for many patients gluten is a trigger and causes general inflammation, and therefore is just part of a healthy diet. The same idea goes for dairy, caffeine, and alcohol. The idea is not to eat foods that are just gluten- or dairy-free, really what we're trying to do is have a patient eat more fruit, vegetables, and healthy meats.

Basic Food Groups to Avoid

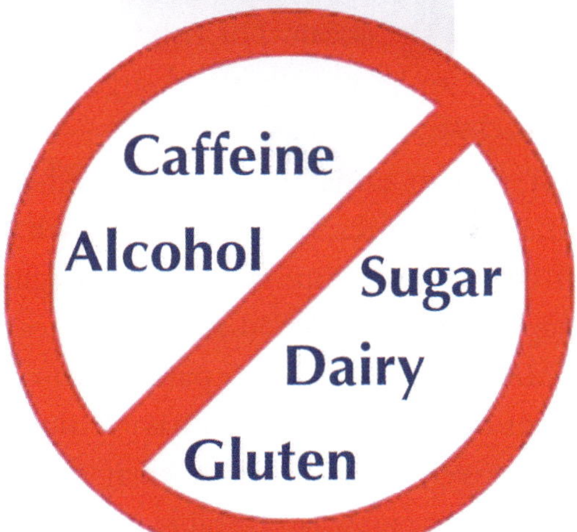

This brings me to the second very important point about migraine diet: blood sugar regulation. If you're unfamiliar with blood sugar regulation, it is the way in which the body moves and stores sugar from food into the blood stream. When you eat, your body absorbs sugar, or glucose, into the bloodstream as fuel for different cells throughout the body. If your blood sugar is too high, you release the hormone insulin. Insulin acts as a key to unlock the cell membrane and allow for glucose to enter various different cells. If your blood sugar gets too low, your body releases glucagon, which causes the liver to convert glycogen into glucose, which is then released into the blood stream to stabilize blood sugar. Your body loves it when blood sugar is stable, like slow rolling waves on the ocean, not rising too high or dipping too low. Your goal is to keep your blood sugar from spiking too high or diving too low.

The easiest way to understand how blood sugar works is by thinking of it like a fire. If you add a bunch of leaves and twigs to the fire it will flare up, but then die right back down. This is what happens to your blood sugar when eating sugars or simple carbohydrates such as bread or pasta. If you put some large branches and logs on the fire, you will have a nice, slow burning fire that stays relatively steady. This is what fats, proteins, and complex carbohydrates (such as vegetables) do your blood sugar. Your body hates large fluctuations in blood sugar and will become more inflamed with larger spikes and dips in blood sugar levels. For example, chronic high levels of blood sugar creates insulin resistance, the basis of diseases such as diabetes or metabolic syndrome. Going in the other direction, low blood sugar is what I call the 'no willpower zone'. When blood sugar is low (hypoglycemia) so is your willpower, so you're more likely to not make a healthy decision.

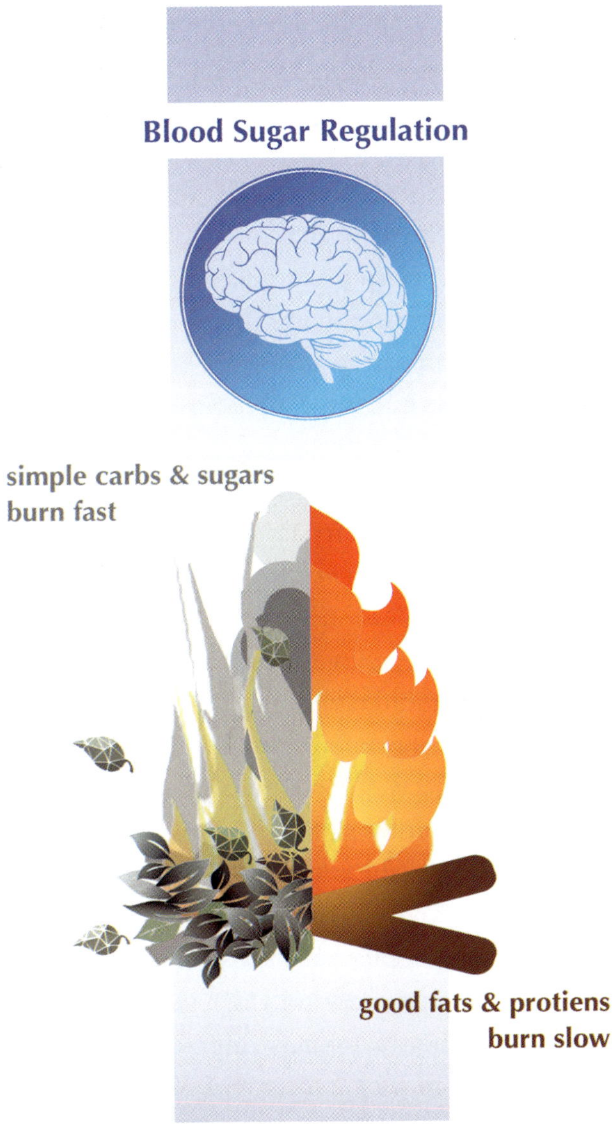
Blood Sugar Regulation
simple carbs & sugars
burn fast
good fats & protiens
burn slow

Think of blood sugar regulation like tending to a campfire. If you throw a bunch of leaves and twigs on the fire it will flare up, but then die down very quickly. That is what happens to your blood sugar when consuming sugars or simple carbohydrates, blood sugar will spike and then decrease quickly, which can cause inflammation. If you throw logs on the fire, they will burn slowly and consistently. This is how good fats, proteins, and complex carbohydrates impact blood sugar.

In order to keep your blood sugar steady, avoid meals with large amounts of sugar or carbohydrates. If you do want to eat something like rice, make sure it is less than 25% of your meal and eat it with some type of fat or protein. Also, try to eat regular, smaller meals every two or three hours. If you want to eat breakfast, lunch, and dinner, just make sure to have a snack in between each meal. Snacks can be as simple as a piece of fruit or a handful of nuts (assuming you're not sensitive to them). Mastering blood sugar regulation is huge dietary component that often gets overlooked in migraine treatment, but it is imperative for a good outcome.

I'll make a quick comment on another dietary consideration for migraine patients. For people that are not having frequent migraines, there is the option to try fasting at some point. If you do decide to do this, I recommend not attempting it without the supervision of a healthcare professional. People with hypoglycemia, for example, run the risk of passing out or having complications with fasting, and therefore should not attempt this approach. The reason for fasting in migraine is primarily for increasing insulin receptor sensitivity. When we are well fed constantly, insulin receptors are frequently bombarded with insulin and therefore become less sensitive to it. Fasting decreases the amount of insulin being released and can reset receptor sensitivity. I personally do not recommend this for my patients, as the people that I see would get markedly worse during the entire fast. Also, most of the research regarding fasting and migraine explains how it induces migraine. While this mechanism makes sense, the idea of fasting with short-term increases in migraine may lead to long-term reduction in migraine if done properly. This is an area of study I'd love to see develop in the near future.

CHAPTER 11

HORMONES & STRESS

Hormonal and stress involvement in migraine has been recognized as long as migraine has been studied. There is a separate type of migraine known as menstrual migraine that accounts for women that only have migraines around their cycle. Many studies also link the fact that patients with higher amounts of stress in their lives tend to have worse outcomes with migraine in both the short and long term (Cha, 2017; Hawkins, 2018). While these two subjects may not seem to be linked at first, if you understand what leads to the creation of stress hormones and sex hormones, you'll find that they are intimately interconnected. You'll also find that the way in which this is currently addressed does not make sense with the pathology of migraine.

When we undergo any type of stress, our body responds by activating the sympathetic nervous system. This is part of the autonomic nervous system that is responsible for the 'fight or flight' response. Part of this response is to release stress hormones into the blood stream in order to increase the capacity for you to respond to danger. This is all regulated through the hypothalamic–pituitary–adrenal (HPA) axis in the brain. The hypothalamus gets feedback from the circulating hormones and sends signals to the pituitary gland to tell it how to respond. The pituitary helps regulate glands like the adrenal or thyroid, and sends signals to tell each gland how much hormone or steroid to produce. The output of the adrenal gland for the fight or flight response is cortisol, a glucocorticosteroid that is distributed throughout the entire body. Cortisol allows the body to respond globally to any perceived danger, such as running away from a predator or saving a child from a dangerous situation.

This is all a normal and necessary response. The problem is that you have a similar release in cortisol whether you're running away from a tiger or taking your chemistry final. The every day stresses of modern life elicit this HPA axis response and can lead to extended periods of increased circulating cortisol. Since this is the hormone that is used to get away from danger, your body will produce it at the expense of other hormones. You can imagine that it's not so important to make sure your sex hormones are balanced if you get mauled by a bear because you didn't have any cortisol reserves. Therefore, people that have extended or intense stressors will 'steal' hormone resources from things like testosterone, estrogen, or progesterone. This is sometimes referred to as 'pregnenolone steal' because pregnenolone is the 'master hormone' that can lead to the production of any other hormone. This concept is somewhat controversial and incomplete, but the big picture idea helps when explaining the basic connection of hormones and migraine to patients. In reality, hormones aren't being 'stolen', rather the HPA axis becomes down-regulated due to prolonged, increased levels of circulating cortisol. This is why our actual treatment for hormonal or nutritional imbalance is based off of the lab testing and is only used when necessary. Many times patients will report that they were tested and have low levels of estrogen or progesterone and are now on estrogen or progesterone supplementation. The rationale makes sense, but I believe they're missing the bigger picture as to why these hormones are out of balance to begin with.

When I start looking at hormones, my first thought goes to where a patient's stress levels are and if other hormones are depleted. Very commonly I will see that the cortisol levels in patients throughout the day is much lower than normal. I often also see lower levels of dehydroepiandrosterone (DHEA), a precursor to testosterone and estrogen. Some research has shown lower DHEA and DHEA/cortisol ratios in migraine patients when compared to controls (Kokavec, 2010). Other papers, however, report that there isn't as much of a difference between cortisol levels in migraine patients vs. controls (Lippi, 2017). As with many areas of migraine research, it's not uncommon to see conflicting data. For me, it all goes back to a very simple principle with migraine patients and how to treat them, which is 'it depends'. This is why we perform comprehensive hormonal testing on patients to see if there is actually something worth working on or if it is not a concern for this particular person.

As far as treating hormonal imbalances, I like to start hormone treatments from the top down. This means that if I see multiple hormones with altered levels, I will supplement with the hormones that can produce all other hormones, such as pregnenolone or DHEA, when indicated. Pregnenolone can turn into any hormone, so if estrogen is low because the patient has been under stress and all of the hormonal resources were going to cortisol, the pregnenolone can go to estrogen if needed. However, if the patient is still undergoing a great amount of stress, the pregnenolone might all be converted to cortisol and leave the low estrogen problem. This is why we also use DHEA, which cannot be converted back into cortisol. This is at a very low dose, depending on the lab results, and it helps the patient to produce some sex hormones, even if they are undergoing a great amount of stress.

While we like to start with the top down approach, there are certain cases that do need some more targeted hormonal support, which is when I may give low dosages of bio-identical progesterone. This is why I won't say that any type of hormone treatment is bad, it's just that it has to be done in this top down order, otherwise we're only addressing the end result and not the reason the imbalance existed in the first place. I tend to find that most migraine patients do great with top down care and we do not have to move on to individual sex hormones.

The interesting thing about this type of treatment is that it was developed primarily for fatigue, weight gain, and female hormone issues, so the protocol is primarily dietary with just a small amount of additional hormones based on lab results. Before I focused on migraine, trying to get patients to stick to the diet was probably the hardest part. Since we are already making dietary changes for migraine specifically, the addition of this protocol into care ends up being simply a few drops of two different hormones. That's it. It's a very simple addition too, since migraine patients understand the importance of diet in their treatment.

Patient Story

Linda

Linda came to see us for her migraines that had intensified over the last few years following a concussion. She had suffered from migraines since she was seven years old, but they had only been occasional. When she came to our office, she had had a migraine 85 times in the last 90 days! She was on cannabis, Triptans, and various other remedies and medications.

Before she even got to the office, her lab work showed that while she had normal levels of estrogen, it was being converted into the harmful 16-OH-E1 metabolite instead of the protective 2-OH-E1 metabolite. She was also not producing enough endogenous glutathione, which is one of the body's natural antioxidants. We made a few tweaks to her diet and added in one more supplement to combat these problems right before she traveled to our office.

We saw her for one week in which she had only one migraine on the first day after a full day of travel. The rest of the week her head pain never made it above a 2/10, and even that was only for a brief period. Her neurological exam was surprisingly good, so we were pushing her mentally and physically the entire week with no flare-ups. She reported that she had not had even two days like this in a row since the concussion, let alone a full week!

STRESS

As discussed earlier in this chapter, an underlying issue that leads to the hormonal dysfunction is chronic stress. The first step is to try to avoid or change any significant stressors in your life. Maybe it's a relationship or friend that causes the problem. It could be an estranged family member you wish you could connect with, or even just animosity with a co-worker that could be improved with a conversation. You may say, "well, I can't escape my job so there's nothing I can do about it". Or, "my family situation is what raises my stress levels and there's nothing I can do about that". It very well may be true, so there are a few things that you can do even if you can't escape your current situation.

The first recommendation that I make to all of my migraine patients is that they should begin some type of mindfulness meditation regimen. Mindfulness has been practiced by many different cultures and religions over thousands of years, but has only recently been studied so that we can understand why it can be so beneficial. For migraine patients, the reason it's so powerful is that it reduces overall stress and decreases your response to stressors. This way, even if your co-worker is being their usual annoying self, your reaction to it is dampened and therefore your output of stress hormones is dampened as well. Having a diminished reaction to daily stressors makes a big difference over time, the same way working out for a day doesn't do a whole lot, but a consistent exercise routine for six months can change you're entire body.

I highly recommend working with a mindfulness practitioner or using a guided mindfulness app or program if you are unfamiliar with the practice. The basic premise is to focus on one thing. It can be a word, a scene, or simply the way that you are breathing. This focus activates a part of the brain known as the default mode network that helps with interception and feelings of contentment.

The natural course for the brain is to focus away from the breath or word onto things like your to-do list or what you're going to make for dinner. This is normal and natural, so once you recognize that your brain is wandering, you simply bring it back to that singular focus. Most people get frustrated when they first begin because they realize how quickly and how often the mind begins to wander. This is okay! The whole point of the practice is not to keep your mind from wandering, it's to recognize when it does and allow yourself to focus back on your breath (or word or scene). Mindfulness will take time to get good at, but research shows that doing about 20 minutes a day is what you want to aim for. That's where the benefits start to be significant. However, if you are getting frustrated and can only do five minutes, start at five minutes and gradually increase until you can get to 20 minutes. I always say that five minutes of mindfulness is better than no minutes of mindfulness.

The second practice that helps keep the stress response under control is high intensity, short duration interval exercise (HIT). A study conducted in 2017 demonstrated that compared to no exercise or moderate exercise, HIT showed a consistent reduction in migraine days (Hanssen 2017). The study also showed an improvement in the patient's arteriolar to venular ratios (A/V ratio), which are an indication of autonomic dysfunction. As we've discussed many times in this book, autonomic dysfunction is one of the main indications that we can test for that indicates migraine. This type of activity increases the body's ability to react to stress appropriately. The same way that a muscle gets stronger as you use it, using this type of 'good stress' strengthens your body's ability to deal with 'bad stress'.

Of course with migraine there is a caveat to this. If the brain and autonomic centers are not very healthy, this type of exercise could actually act as a stressor and increase the probability of a migraine. Think of it like training the 80-year old man in chapter 8 for a marathon. If he hasn't run in 20 years, starting with a 15-mile run is probably not going to end well. However, if he starts with a half mile and keeps increasing over time, eventually he can run the full 15 miles. The same goes for this type of activity and migraine. If you find that exercise is a trigger, it doesn't mean that it's bad for you, it means you're doing too much of a good thing. You may need to start with simple (but not easy) isometric exercises such as planks or wall sits. You can then begin light cardio such as an elliptical machine, bike, or simply walking. We use this type of graded increase in activity with just about every aspect of migraine treatment.

Combining mindfulness meditation and high intensity interval training (HIT) is a great way to introduce control over your migraines when you're stuck in situations that you may not be able to get out of at the time. One consistent 'miracle' I see with migraine patients is the fact that they magically improve when they go on a nice relaxing vacation. So short of prescribing permanent vacations (which, trust me, I wish I could do), these activities are your best shot at dealing with the day-to-day stressors that 'fill up the bucket' and make migraines more likely.

CHAPTER 12

MUSCULOSKELETAL STRESS

"You have to go see my chiropractor, she is a miracle worker and she'll cure your migraines like she did for me!" "You have to go see my acupuncturist, he fixed me up after a few treatments and I'm healed!" "My massage therapist is God's gift to migraine sufferers, you have to go see them!"

If you've had a migraine for more than two minutes, you've undoubtedly heard this from at least 28 people, and before I go any further I want to make it clear that I think ALL of these types of treatments are great and worth exploring. However, if one of them was the cure-all for migraine, there would only be one modality that consistently heals migraine, which just isn't the case. If migraine was just caused by fixated joints, there's no reason why massage wouldn't help. If dysfunction in the body's Chi was the cause of migraine, you'd never have to see a chiropractor. The point is that the research supports chiropractic, acupuncture, massage, trigger point therapy, and a variety of other musculoskeletal treatments for migraine. Why?

One thing that all of these treatments have in common is that they work on different sensory pathways that project to different areas of the brain. For example, a chiropractor activates muscle spindle receptors deep in the body close to the spine. These muscle spindles fire to the ipsilateral (same side) cerebellum, and eventually to the contralateral (opposite) cortex. We've seen in research that there is also activation of the prefrontal cortices following spinal manipulative therapy (SMT) (Lelic, 2016). Acupuncture works primarily on c-fibers and has been shown to help modulate the abnormal brainstem activity in the trigeminocervical nucleus (Li, 2017). Massage gives more feedback to the superficial muscles and cerebellum. The reason that these modalities can all cause significant changes is due to the fact that the parts of the brain they project to are integrators. These are areas that take in various types of information in order to allow the brain to make sense of the world. If the primary dysfunction in a migraineur is in the cerebellum, massage or chiropractic might be effective. If it's in the prefrontal areas, chiropractic alone might be more helpful. If it's primarily in the brainstem, any technique could be helpful depending on the side or stimulation and the part of the body stimulated.

The most important aspect to remember is that all of these methods are helping to stabilize the nervous system and relieve increased musculoskeletal stress. This helps to reduce the probability that someone will experience a migraine, but it is only one piece of the puzzle. If this person's main bucket filler is musculoskeletal stress, then chiropractic or acupuncture or massage will seem like a miracle cure, which is awesome! The only downside is it leads each individual practitioner into a false sense of success where they see people getting better with what they do, but if someone doesn't get better there's no next step.

Here's what typically happens. If someone starts having migraine and their main trigger is musculoskeletal, they may see a chiropractor. If it helps, and it was their first stop, both the patient and the chiropractor would assume that chiropractic was the cure for migraine. If that same person had already tried nutrition, acupuncture, and medications, and then finally gets to the chiropractor and it helps, both the doctor and patient are going to think that it was obviously because chiropractic cures migraine.

Now let's look at another person who has equal amounts of stress from nutrition, musculoskeletal problems, and hormonal issues. If they start by addressing the hormonal and nutritional components and they still experience migraine, then they try a chiropractor and it gets better, they'll both think that chiropractic was the solution. If that same patient was to try chiropractic first, they wouldn't have great success and the doctor would be disappointed but not know why this person didn't respond as well. However, because they already fixed the musculoskeletal problems, when this patient gets to the nutritionist or hormone specialist they'll get better and attribute it the nutrition and hormones and not the chiropractor. This logic can apply to any practitioner, I simply used chiropractic for consistency. Hopefully this gives you an idea why many practitioners (medical doctors, nutritionists, chiropractic doctors, acupuncturists, massage therapists, etc.) can have many successes with migraine patients, but the people that have dysfunction in multiple areas end up bouncing around from doctor to doctor with no answers.

This is the most consistent story that I hear when I talk to people from all over the world. They've tried literally every type of treatment you can imagine and still have consistent migraines. Again, it's not that any of those treatments weren't good, they were probably great for them, but no one individual practitioner put all the pieces together to fully address the altered brain state they are dealing with. This is most common with chronic migraine patients, of which there are over 4 million in the US alone. If we were able to get everyone thinking about migraine in the same way, we could save millions of people years and years of their lives from being afflicted with severe disability.

CHAPTER 13

WHERE DO WE GO FROM HERE?

If you've made it this far, hopefully by now you have a strong and profound understanding of how migraine actually works and how to go about looking for answers. Due to more and more research coming out about neuromodulation and the idea of brain stimulation with migraine, there has been a host of new products and procedures on the market. Many of them are hit or miss, but not detrimental to health, meaning that they are worth a shot and if they don't work just stop using it. With more and more options for migraine treatment hitting the market every week, what can we do better, both as patients and doctors, to help reverse and manage this debilitating condition?

There are a few main avenues I believe should be explored further to get a better handle on migraine. The first and foremost is proper diagnosis. For example, many of the studies that talk about differences in gray matter in the brain are using functional magnetic resonance imaging (fMRI). The studies take a large sample of migraine patients and then find differences in gray matter volume compared to non-migraine patients. The next step would be using individual fMRI studies to see if these areas are altered in all migraine patients, or if only certain areas are altered in individual patients. Based on my clinical experience, I would expect that you would find gray matter alterations in a few of the areas already identified in research, but not all. Each person should be able to have imaging done, know what parts of the brain have altered gray matter, and then be prescribed therapies targeted at that part of the brain to increase the stability of the area.

There also needs to be a consensus as to what is 'true migraine'. Currently, the criteria allows for many types of headache to be classified as migraine. We need to have consistent, objective criteria that identify migraine patients vs. those that have headaches that are not adequately or better explained by other conditions (as mentioned in chapter 2 I would suggest 'migraine-like headache disorders'). This would not only help patients, but it would also help researches to be more specific about the type of patients being used for research, therefore making outcomes more accurate. In my opinion, it is very unlikely that you find true migraine without autonomic dysfunction, so testing that involves autonomic evaluation should be pursued as possible objective diagnostic criteria.

For me, I would also like to see research that confirms the theory that we are able to change the excitability of the pools of neurons to which we are stimulating. Currently, we are only able to extrapolate that as patients are improving and their resting membrane potential is stabilizing. A consistent, measurable way to evaluate these changes could be instrumental in the future care of migraine in that it would allow us to determine exactly how much stimulation is appropriate for each patient. It would also give feedback as to whether a therapy that should work or stimulate a specific part of the brain is actually working effectively.

This is part of why I'm currently teaching a post-doctoral course specifically on migraine. Not head pain, not headaches, not head and face pain disorders – just migraine. I want to get input and feedback from as many different practitioners as possible so that we can all be on the same page about what's going on with migraine. As you can hopefully see by this point, the condition is very different from any other type of headache or pain pathology. This book is basically a very abbreviated version of the material that I am teaching in this course to other doctors. My goal with the course is to have doctors from all different professions become experts in migraine so they can apply their specialty to their treatment of the condition, but also be knowledgeable enough to know when and where to send patients when they need other forms of care.

My hope is that this book sparks the curiosity of people from all backgrounds and specialties. Maybe a doctor that specializes in gene therapy thinks of a new way to target the ion channels associated with migraine. Maybe a physical therapist creates a migraine exercise progression program to help people exercise that previously shouldn't exercise because it may cause their symptoms to flare up. Maybe a medical doctor finds a more effective way to identify which migraine medications will adversely affect an individual patient, so they don't have all of the negative side effects that are usually experienced. There might also be a patient out there that has lost hope about ever having a normal life, that finally understands what's going on and how they may begin moving down their migraine spectrum toward fewer and fewer attacks. Whatever it was that led you to read this book, I hope it helps move us all toward the ultimate goal of mastering migraine.

Bibliography

1. Amin FM, Asghar MS, Hougaard A, Hansen AE, Larsen VA, de Koning PJ, Larsson HB, Olesen J, Ashina M. Magnetic resonance angiography of intracranial and extracranial arteries in patients with spontaneous migraine without aura: a cross-sectional study. Lancet Neurol. 2013 May; 12(5):454-61. doi: 10.1016/S1474-4422(13)70067-X. Epub 2013 Apr 9. PubMed PMID: 23578775.
2. Anzalone AJ, Blueitt D, Case T, McGuffin T, Pollard K, Garrison JC, Jones MT, Pavur R, Turner S, Oliver JM. A Positive Vestibular/Ocular Motor Screening (VOMS) is Associated with Increased Recovery Time After Sports-Related Concussion in Youth and Adolescent Athletes. Am J Sports Med. 2017 Feb; 45(2):474-479. doi: 10.1177/0363546516668624. Epub 2016 Oct 28. PubMed PMID: 27789472.
3. Avnon Y, Nitzan M, Sprecher E, Rogowski Z, Yarnitsky D. Autonomic asymmetry in migraine: augmented parasympathetic activation in left unilateral migraineurs. Brain. 2004 Sep; 127(Pt 9):2099-108. Epub 2004 Jul 28. PubMed PMID: 15282213.
4. Aymoz D, Wosika V, Durandau E, Pelet S. Real-time quantification of protein expression at the single-cell level via dynamic protein synthesis translocation reporters. Nat Commun. 2016 Apr 21; 7:11304. doi: 10.1038/ncomms11304. PubMed PMID: 27098003; PubMed Central PMCID: PMC4844680.

5. Balci B, Şenyuva N, Akdal G. Definition of Balance and Cognition Related to Disability Levels in Vestibular Migraine Patients. Noro Psikiyatr Ars. 2018 Mar 19; 55(1):9-14. doi: 10.29399/npa.12617. eCollection 2018 Mar. PubMed PMID: 30042635; PubMed Central PMCID: PMC6045802.
6. Bernetti L, Pellegrino C, Corbelli I, Caproni S, Eusebi P, Faralli M, Ricci G, Calabresi P, Sarchielli P. Subclinical vestibular dysfunction in migraineurs without vertigo: a clinical study. Acta Neurol Scand. 2018 Apr 16. doi: 10.1111/ane.12941. (Epub ahead of print) PubMed PMID: 29658983.
7. Bonafede M, Cai Q, Cappell K, Kim G, Sapra SJ, Shah N, Widnell K, Winner P, Desai P. Factors Associated with Direct Health Care Costs Among Patients with Migraine. J Manage Care Spec Pharm. 2017 Nov; 23(11):1169-1176. doi: 10.18553/jmcp.2017.23.11.1169. PubMed PMID: 29083975.
8. Burch R, Rizzoli P, Loder E. The Prevalence and Impact of Migraine and Severe Headache in the United States: Figures and Trends From Government Health Studies. Headache. 2018 Apr; 58(4):496-505. doi: 10.1111/head.13281. Epub 2018 Mar 12. PubMed PMID: 29527677.
9. Cai X, Shi X, Zhang X, Zhang A, Zheng M, Fang Y. The association between brain-derived neurotrophic factor gene polymorphism and migraine: a meta-analysis. J Headache Pain. 2017 Dec; 18(1):13. doi: 10.1186/s10194-017-0725-2. Epub 2017 Feb 2. Review. PubMed PMID: 28150221; PubMed Central PMCID: PMC5289130.
10. Carrera E, Tononi G. Diaschisis: past, present, future. Brain. 2014 Sep; 137(Pt 9):2408-22. doi: 10.1093/brain/awu101. Epub 2014 May 28. Review. PubMed PMID: 24871646.
11. Carrick FR, Clark JF, Pagnacco G, Antonucci MM, Hankir A, Zaman R, Oggero E. Head-Eye Vestibular Motion Therapy Affects the Mental and Physical Health of Severe Chronic Postconcussion Patients. Front Neurol. 2017 Aug 22; 8:414. doi: 10.3389/

fneur.2017.00414. eCollection 2017. PubMed PMID: 28878731; PubMed Central PMCID: PMC5572417.

12. Cassidy P, Jones K. A study of inter-arm blood pressure differences in primary care. J Hum Hypertens. 2001 Aug; 15(8):519-22. PubMed PMID: 11494088.
13. Cha MJ, Kim BK, Moon HS, Ahn JY, Oh K, Kim JY, Kim BS, Sohn JH, Chung JM, Song TJ, Kim J, Seo JG, Chu MK, Cho SJ. Stress is Associated with Poor Outcome of Acute Treatment for Chronic Migraine: a Multicenter Study. Pain Med. 2017 Nov 2. doi: 10.1093/pm/pnx269. (Epub ahead of print) PubMed PMID: 29106663.
14. Chong CD, Plasencia JD, Frakes DH, Schwedt TJ. Structural alterations of the brainstem in migraine. Neuroimage Clin. 2016 Nov 2; 13:223-227. doi: 10.1016/j.nicl.2016.10.023. eCollection 2017. PubMed PMID: 28003961; PubMed Central PMCID: PMC5157793.
15. De Marchis ML, Guadagni F, Silvestris E, Lovero D, Della-Morte D, Ferroni P, Barbanti P, Palmirotta R. Genetic bases of the nutritional approach to migraine. Crit Rev Food Sci Nutr. 2018 Mar 8:1-13. doi: 10.1080/10408398.2018.1450215. (Epub ahead of print) PubMed PMID: 29517920.
16. Deng Y, Huang J, Zhang H, Zhu X, Gong Q. Association of expression of DRD2 rs1800497 polymorphism with migraine risk in Han Chinese individuals. J Pain Res. 2018 Apr 12; 11:763-769. doi: 10.2147/JPR.S151350. eCollection 2018. PubMed PMID: 29695928; PubMed Central PMCID: PMC5905461.
17. Dhifallah S, Lancaster E, Merrill S, Leroudier N, Mantegazza M, Cestèle S. Gain of Function for the SCN1A/hNa(v)1.1-L1670W Mutation Responsible for Familial Hemiplegic Migraine. Front Mol Neurosci. 2018 Jul 9; 11:232. doi: 10.3389/fnmol.2018.00232. eCollection 2018. PubMed PMID: 30038559; PubMed Central PMCID: PMC6046441.
18. Drummond PD. Photophobia and autonomic responses to facial pain in migraine. Brain. 1997 Oct; 120 (Pt 10):1857-64. PubMed PMID: 9365375.

19. Eising E, A Datson N, van den Maagdenberg AM, Ferrari MD. Epigenetic mechanisms in migraine: a promising avenue? BMC Med. 2013 Feb 4; 11:26. doi: 10.1186/1741-7015-11-26. Review. PubMed PMID: 23379668; PubMed Central PMCID: PMC3584973.
20. Erdal K. Neuropsychological testing for sports-related concussion: how athletes can sandbag their baseline testing without detection. Arch Clin Neuropsychol. 2012 Aug; 27(5):473-9. doi: 10.1093/arclin/acs050. Epub 2012 Jun 8. PubMed PMID: 22684033.
21. Eren OE, Ruscheweyh R, Schankin C, Schöberl F, Straube A. The cold pressor test in interictal migraine patients – different parasympathetic pupillary response indicates dysbalance of the cranial autonomic nervous system. BMC Neurol. 2018 Apr 16; 18(1):41. doi: 10.1186/s12883-018-1043-2. PubMed PMID: 29661162; PubMed Central PMCID: PMC5901875.
22. Formeister EJ, Rizk HG, Kohn MA, Sharon JD. The Epidemiology of Vestibular Migraine: a Population-based Survey Study. Otol Neurotol. 2018 Jul 16. doi: 10.1097/MAO.0000000000001900. (Epub ahead of print) PubMed PMID: 30020261.
23. Fotherby MD, Panayiotou B, Potter JF. Age-related differences in simultaneous interarm blood pressure measurements. Postgrad Med J. 1993 Mar; 69(809): 194-6. PubMed PMID: 8497433; PubMed Central PMCID: PMC2399734.
24. Goadsby PJ, Holland PR, Martins-Oliveira M, Hoffmann J, Schankin C, Akerman S. Pathophysiology of Migraine: a Disorder of Sensory Processing. Physiol Rev. 2017 Apr; 97(2):553-622.
25. González-Hernández A, Marichal-Cancino BA, Maassen-VanDenBrink A, Villalón CM. Side effects associated with current and prospective antimigraine pharmacotherapies. Expert Opin Drug Metab Toxicol. 2018 Jan; 14(1):25-41. doi: 10.1080/17425255.2018.1416097. Epub 2017 Dec 15. Review. PubMed PMID: 29226741.
26. Grool AM, Aglipay M, Momoli F, Meehan WP 3rd, Freedman SB, Yeates KO, Gravel J, Gagnon I, Boutis K, Meeuwisse W,

Barrowman N, Ledoux AA, Osmond MH, Zemek R; Pediatric Emergency Research Canada (PERC) Concussion Team. Association Between Early Participation in Physical Activity Following Acute Concussion and Persistent Postconcussive Symptoms in Children and Adolescents. JAMA. 2016 Dec 20; 316(23):2504-2514. doi: 10.1001/jama.2016.17396. PubMed PMID: 27997652.

27. Grossman A, Prokupetz A, Gordon B, Morag-Koren N, Grossman E. Inter-arm blood pressure differences in young, healthy patients. J Clin Hypertens (Greenwich). 2013 Aug; 15(8):575-8. doi: 10.1111/jch.12125. Epub 2013 May 10. PubMed PMID: 23889720.
28. Hanssen H, Minghetti A, Magon S, Rossmeissl A, Rasenack M, Papadopoulou A, Klenk C, Faude O, Zahner L, Sprenger T, Donath L. Effects of different endurance exercise modalities on migraine days and cerebrovascular health in episodic migraineurs: a randomized controlled trial. Scand J Med Sci Sports. 2017 Nov 21. doi: 10.1111/sms.13023. (Epub ahead of print) PubMed PMID: 29161767.
29. Hawkins JL, Moore NJ, Miley D, Durham PL. Secondary traumatic stress increases expression of proteins implicated in peripheral and central sensitization of trigeminal neurons. Brain Res. 2018 May 15; 1687:162-172. doi: 10.1016/j.brainres.2018.03.003. Epub 2018 Mar 6. PubMed PMID: 29522721; PubMed Central PMCID: PMC5882570.
30. Hebestreit JM, May A. Topiramate modulates trigeminal pain processing in thalamo-cortical networks in humans after single dose administration. PLoS One. 2017 Oct 9; 12(10):e0184406. doi: 10.1371/journal.pone.0184406. eCollection 2017. PubMed PMID: 28991914; PubMed Central PMCID: PMC5633146.
31. Hu W, Guo J, Chen N, Guo J, He L. A meta-analysis of voxel-based morphometric studies on migraine. Int J Clin Exp Med. 2015 Mar 15;8(3):4311-9. eCollection 2015. PubMed PMID: 26064347; PubMed Central PMCID: PMC4443181.
32. Kokavec A, Crebbin SJ. Sugar alters the level of serum insulin and plasma glucose and the serum cortisol: DHEAS ratio in female

migraine sufferers. Appetite. 2010 Dec; 55(3):582-8. doi: 10.1016/j.appet.2010.09.007. Epub 2010 Sep 21. PubMed PMID: 20851729.

33. Latham PW. On Nervous or Sick-Headache. Cambridge, UK: Deighton, Bell and Co., 1873.

34. Lawrence DW, Richards D, Comper P, Hutchison MG. Earlier time to aerobic exercise is associated with faster recovery following acute sport concussion. PLoS One. 2018 Apr 18; 13(4):e0196062. doi: 10.1371/journal.pone.0196062. eCollection 2018. PubMed PMID: 29668716; PubMed Central PMCID: PMC5905975.

35. Lee MJ, Choi HA, Choi H, Chung CS. Caffeine discontinuation improves acute migraine treatment: a prospective clinic-based study. J Headache Pain. 2016 Dec; 17(1):71. doi: 10.1186/s10194-016-0662-5. Epub 2016 Aug 5. PubMed PMID: 27492448; PubMed Central PMCID: PMC4975726.

36. Lee SH, Jeong SH, Kim JS, Kim HJ, Choi KD, Choi JH, Oh SY, Park JY, Kim DU, Kim BK. Effect of Prophylactic Medication on Associated Dizziness and Motion Sickness in Migraine. Otol Neurotol. 2018 Jan; 39(1):e45-e51. doi:10.1097/MAO.0000000000001628. PubMed PMID: 29227453.

37. Lelic D, Niazi IK, Holt K, Jochumsen M, Dremstrup K, Yielder P, Murphy B, Drewes AM, Haavik H. Manipulation of Dysfunctional Spinal Joints Affects Sensorimotor Integration in the Prefrontal Cortex: A Brain Source Localization Study. Neural Plast. 2016;2016:3704964. doi: 10.1155/2016/3704964. Epub 2016 Mar 7. PubMed PMID: 27047694; PubMed Central PMCID: PMC4800094.

38. Li Z, Zeng F, Yin T, Lan L, Makris N, Jorgenson K, Guo T, Wu F, Gao Y, Dong M, Liu M, Yang J, Li Y, Gong Q, Liang F, Kong J. Acupuncture modulates the abnormal brainstem activity in migraine without aura patients. Neuroimage Clin. 2017 May 22; 15:367-375. doi: 10.1016/j.nicl.2017.05.013. eCollection 2017. PubMed PMID: 28580293; PubMed Central PMCID: PMC5447510.

39. Lippi G, Mattiuzzi C. Cortisol and migraine: a systematic literature review. Agri. 2017 Jul; 29(3):95-99. doi: 10.5505/agri.2017.25348. PubMed PMID: 29039159.
40. Lipton RB, Diener HC, Robbins MS, Garas SY, Patel K. Caffeine in the management of patients with headache. J Headache Pain. 2017 Oct 24; 18(1):107. doi: 10.1186/s10194-017-0806-2. Review. PubMed PMID: 29067618; PubMed Central PMCID: PMC5655397.
41. Liveing E. On Megrim, Sick-Headache, and Some Allied Disorders. A Contribution to the Pathology of Nerve-Storms. London: Arts & Boeve Nijmegen, 1873.
42. Majerske CW, Mihalik JP, Ren D, Collins MW, Reddy CC, Lovell MR, Wagner AK. Concussion in sports: post-concussive activity levels, symptoms, and neurocognitive performance. J Athl Train. 2008 May-Jun; 43(3):265-74. doi: 10.4085/1062-6050-43.3.265. PubMed PMID: 18523563; PubMed Central PMCID: PMC2386420.
43. Martin U, Holder R, Hodgkinson J, McManus R. Inter-arm blood pressure differences compared with ambulatory monitoring: a manifestation of the 'white-coat' effect? Br J Gen Pract. 2013 Feb; 63(607):e97-103. doi: 10.3399/bjgp13X663055. Erratum in: Br J Gen Pract. 2013 May; 63(610):240. PubMed PMID: 23561681; PubMed Central PMCID: PMC3553646.
44. Mehlsen J, Wiinberg N. Inter-arm difference in blood pressure: reproducibility and association with peripheral vascular disease. Int J Vasc Med. 2014; 2014:841542. doi: 10.1155/2014/841542. Epub 2014 Jan 29. PubMed PMID: 24616810; PubMed Central PMCID: PMC3927742.
45. Mirza AF, Mo J, Holt JL, Kairalla JA, Heft MW, Ding M, Ahn AH. Is there a relationship between throbbing pain and arterial pulsations? J Neurosci. 2012 May 30; 32(22):7572-6. doi: 10.1523/JNEUROSCI.0193-12.2012. PubMed PMID: 22649235; PubMed Central PMCID: PMC3376713.

46. Moulton EA, Becerra L, Johnson A, Burstein R, Borsook D. Altered hypothalamic functional connectivity with autonomic circuits and the locus coeruleus in migraine. PLoS One. 2014 Apr 17; 9(4):e95508. doi: 10.1371/journal.pone.0095508. eCollection 2014. PubMed PMID: 24743801; PubMed Central PMCID: PMC3990690.
47. Mucha A, Collins MW, Elbin RJ, Furman JM, Troutman-Enseki C, DeWolf RM, Marchetti G, Kontos AP. A Brief Vestibular/Ocular Motor Screening (VOMS) assessment to evaluate concussions: preliminary findings. Am J Sports Med. 2014 Oct; 42(10):2479-86. doi: 10.1177/0363546514543775. Epub 2014 Aug 8. PubMed PMID: 25106780; PubMed Central PMCID: PMC4209316.
48. Pan Q, Zhang Y, Long T, He W, Zhang S, Fan Y, Zhou J. Diagnosis of Vertigo and Dizziness Syndromes in a Neurological Outpatient Clinic. Eur Neurol. 2018 May 24; 79(5-6):287-294. doi: 10.1159/000489639. (Epub ahead of print) PubMed PMID: 29794430.
49. Pelzer N, Louter MA, van Zwet EW, Nyholt DR, Ferrari MD, van den Maagdenberg AM, Haan J, Terwindt GM. Linking migraine frequency with family history of migraine. Cephalalgia. 2018 Jan 1:333102418783295. doi: 10.1177/0333102418783295. (Epub ahead of print) PubMed PMID: 29911421.
50. Piovesan EJ, et al. Neuropsiquiatr. 2008 Mar; 66(1):77-9. Episodic migraine associated with postural orthostatic tachycardia syndrome and vasovagal syncope: migraine triggers neuromediated syncope. D, Silberstein S.
51. Rahmann A, Wienecke T, Hansen JM, Fahrenkrug J, Olesen J, Ashina M. Vasoactive intestinal peptide causes marked cephalic vasodilation, but does not induce migraine. Cephalalgia. 2008 Mar; 28(3):226-36. doi: 10.1111/j.1468-2982.2007.01497.x. PubMed PMID: 18254893.
52. Rauschel V, Straube A, Süß F, Ruscheweyh R. Responsiveness of the autonomic nervous system during paced breathing and mental stress in migraine patients. J Headache Pain. 2015; 16:82.

doi: 10.1186/s10194-015-0567-8. Epub 2015 Sep 16. PubMed PMID: 26377932; PubMed Central PMCID: PMC4573080.

53. Scher AI, Stewart WF, Lipton RB. Caffeine as a risk factor for chronic daily headache: a population-based study. Neurology. 2004 Dec 14; 63(11):2022-7. PubMed PMID: 15596744.
54. Schwartz, James H. *Principles of Neural Science*. Edited by Eric R. Kandel and Sarah Mack, 5th ed., McGraw-Hill Medical, 2013. p. 1071, 1025.
55. Schwarz G, Anzalone N, Baldoli C, Impellizzeri M, Minicucci F, Comi G, Colombo B. Pediatric sporadic hemiplegic migraine (ATP1A2 gene): a case report and brief literature review. Neurol Sci. 2018 Jun;39(Suppl 1):69-71. doi: 10.1007/s10072-018-3405-3. PubMed PMID: 29904856.
56. Thompson-Harvey A, Mikulec AA. Total caloric eye speed in patients with vestibular migraine. Am J Otolaryngol. 2017 Nov 14. pii: S0196-0709(17)30610-5. doi: 10.1016/j.amjoto.2017.11.007. (Epub ahead of print) PubMed PMID: 29169953.
57. van der Hoeven NV, Lodestijn S, Nanninga S, van Montfrans GA, van den Born BJ. Simultaneous compared with sequential blood pressure measurement results in smaller inter-arm blood pressure differences. J Clin Hypertens (Greenwich). 2013 Nov; 15(11):839-44. doi: 10.1111/jch.12203. Epub 2013 Sep 19. PubMed PMID: 24102851.
58. Vuralli D, Yildirim F, Akcali DT, Ilhan MN, Goksu N, Bolay H. Visual and Postural Motion-Evoked Dizziness Symptoms are Predominant in Vestibular Migraine Patients. Pain Med. 2017 Jul 13. doi: 10.1093/pm/pnx182. (Epub ahead of print) PubMed PMID: 29017000.
59. Wallasch TM, Beckmann P, Kropp P. Cerebrovascular reactivity during the Valsalva maneuver in migraine, tension-type headache, and medication overuse headache. Funct Neurol. 2011 Oct-Dec; 26(4):223-7. PubMed PMID: 22364943; PubMed Central PMCID: PMC3814561.

60. Wessman M, Terwindt GM, Kaunisto MA, Palotie A, Ophoff RA. Migraine: a complex genetic disorder. Lancet Neurol. 2007 Jun; 6(6):521-32. Review. PubMed PMID: 17509487.
61. Yan J, Dussor G. Ion channels and migraine. Headache. 2014 Apr; 54(4):619-39.doi: 10.1111/head.12323. Review. PubMed PMID: 24697223; PubMed Central PMCID: PMC4005924.
62. Yorke AM, Smith L, Babcock M, Alsalaheen B. Validity and Reliability of the Vestibular/Ocular Motor Screening and Associations with Common Concussion Screening Tools. Sports Health. 2017 Mar/Apr; 9(2):174-180. doi: 10.1177/1941738116678411. Epub 2016 Nov 11. PubMed PMID: 27834667; PubMed Central PMCID: PMC5349391.
63. Zebenholzer K, Gall W, Wöber C. Use and overuse of Triptans in Austria – a survey based on nationwide healthcare claims data. J Headache Pain. 2018 May 18; 19(1):34. doi: 10.1186/s10194-018-0864-0. PubMed PMID: 29777424; PubMed Central PMCID: PMC5959824.

ABOUT THE AUTHOR

Dr. Adam Harcourt is the owner of Imagine X Functional Neurology, with office locations in Beverly Hills and Santa Barbara, CA. He is a Fellow of the American College of Functional Neurology (FACFN), Fellow of the American Board of Vestibular Rehabilitation (FABVR), Diplomate of the American Chiropractic Neurology Board (DACNB), and a fourth generation Doctor of Chiropractic. Dr. Harcourt is also an Associate Professor of Clinical Neurology at Carrick Institute for Graduate Studies, where he travels both domestically and internationally instructing doctors from around the world.

Dr. Harcourt has developed his novel Migraine and Concussion treatment programs based on the latest research, his years of experience seeing patients, and his passion for finding root causes and correcting them. He has become the go-to doctor for these conditions, and his treatment programs bring patients to his California offices from literally around the world.

Dr. Harcourt has also created a 150-hour post-doctoral program, also titled "*Mastering Migraine*", with which he instructs doctors from all different backgrounds from around the world.

Dr. Harcourt is also dedicated to giving back and has served on the Board of Directors at Jodi House Brain Injury Support Center in Santa Barbara, CA, for many years and was Board President from 2017-2018.

Dr. Harcourt has presented multiple abstracts on Migraine, Concussion, Dysautonomia, and Multiple Sclerosis at research symposiums over the past several years. He was a speaker at the International Symposium of Clinical Neuroscience (ISCN) on Migraine in 2018, and a presenter and chair at the Neurological Disorders Symposium (NDS) on his treatment of Migraine in 2019. He is also a sought-after speaker and has spoken at many different events across the U.S. on Migraine and Concussion treatment and diagnosis, podcasts, television interviews, and more.

As the title implies, mastering migraine, is a continual process that changes every day. It's not that we will never master migraine, it's that the mastery will always be improving. To keep up with research breakthroughs, book signings, interviews, helpful tips, and Dr. Harcourt's speaking schedule, please check out www.adamharcourt.com.